"An endearing read...thanks to vibrant, witty storytelling, a second chance at love, and the hovering hope of a happy ending."
—*PEOPLE*

"A straight-out-of-a-movie memoir."
—*PARADE*

"Funny, poignant, and sometimes magical."
—*ASSOCIATED PRESS*

"A heart-wrenching tale of second chances at life and love."
—*TIME*

"Uplifting... A fun and rewarding read."
—*BOSTON GLOBE*

"Radiant... Readers will be swept away by this triumphant story."
—*PUBLISHERS WEEKLY*

W9-CHT-212

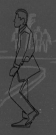
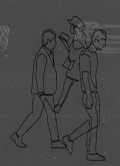
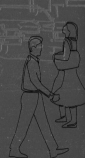

Acclaim for Delia Ephron's

Left on Tenth

"Only someone with a heart of stone could resist the charms of Delia Ephron's tender, moving story of late-life love and illness. Ephron writes with singular transparency of her treatment for leukemia—the same disease that killed her sister seven years earlier—and the unbearable terror and pain she suffered. But she is at heart a writer naturally drawn to light who finds joy and humor even in life's darkest corners. This wonderful memoir is an ode to the enduring power of love and friendship."

—Joanna Rakoff, author of *My Salinger Year*

"This endearing read is anything but depressing thanks to vibrant, witty storytelling, a second chance at love, and the hovering hope of a happy ending right out of a movie."

—*People*

"Ephron should be called the Queen of Second Chances, and long may she reign...Her endurance is nothing short of mind-boggling, her survival to tell the tale even more miraculous...Ephron's account of triumphing over life's greatest challenges is itself a tour de force."

—*Booklist*

"Ephron masterfully and hilariously reminds us that there is always more life to be found just around the corner. A powerful, beautiful, life-affirming testament to hope and meaning in the darkest hour. Somehow it felt like the answers to all the big questions were hiding in the text. Like any decent existentialist and searcher, I couldn't put it down and finished it in one sitting."

—Natasha Lyonne, writer, director, and actor

"This funny, poignant, and sometimes magical memoir is an open-eyed look at later life and what Ephron calls the left turns that can be perilous or wondrous."

—Anita Snow, Associated Press

"Delia Ephron is the voice of our times and a master craftsman of the written word. If you are looking for a book that tells you the truth about love, marriage, friendship, family, creativity, loss, redemption, and your internet provider, look no further. Ephron soars on the page, and takes us with her."

—Adriana Trigiani, author of
The Good Left Undone

"Delia Ephron knows how to grip a reader with plot twists and punchy prose."   —Julia M. Klein, *The Forward*

"*Left on Tenth* is less the story of a woman losing a husband than it is that of a woman falling in love again at age seventy-two . . . Ephron's story is inspiring for all of us out there whose romantic lives or longings will never be the stuff of a big-box-office romantic comedy . . . If there's such a thing as a feel-good memoir, this is it."

—Joyce Maynard, *New York Times Book Review*

"Radiant...Readers will be swept away by this triumphant story."
—*Publishers Weekly*

"Oh, huge-hearted Delia Ephron! I loved this book. It's a memoir about grief and illness, but it's also basically a love letter to her people, and it's a gorgeous one. Because here is someone who chooses joy over and over again—who chooses friendship and love, like a fountain of gratitude that turns despair into a glittery, rainbow-scattering spray of light. Her lucky friends! Forgive yourself for wishing you were one of them."
—Catherine Newman, author of
Catastrophic Happiness

"Ephron's memoir is a heart-wrenching tale of second chances at life and love."
—*Time*

"Delia Ephron's stunning memoir will make you believe in love again, and also in miracles. And it's so very, very funny."
—Sarah Dunn, author of *The Arrangement*

ALSO BY DELIA EPHRON

Novels
Siracusa
The Lion Is In
Big City Eyes
Hanging Up

Nonfiction
Sister Mother Husband Dog (Etc.)
Funny Sauce

Humor
How to Eat Like a Child
Teenage Romance
Do I Have to Say Hello?

Young Adult
Frannie in Pieces
The Girl with the Mermaid Hair

Children's
The Girl Who Changed the World
Santa and Alex
My Life (and Nobody Else's)

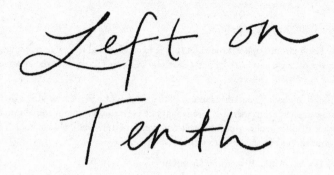

Left on Tenth

A Second Chance at Life

A Memoir

Delia Ephron

BACK BAY BOOKS

Little, Brown and Company

New York   Boston   London

Copyright © 2022 by Delia Ephron

Hachette Book Group supports the right to free expression and the value of copyright. The purpose of copyright is to encourage writers and artists to produce the creative works that enrich our culture.

The scanning, uploading, and distribution of this book without permission is a theft of the author's intellectual property. If you would like permission to use material from the book (other than for review purposes), please contact permissions@hbgusa.com. Thank you for your support of the author's rights.

Back Bay Books / Little, Brown and Company
Hachette Book Group
1290 Avenue of the Americas, New York, NY 10104
littlebrown.com

Originally published in hardcover by Little, Brown and Company, April 2022
First Back Bay paperback edition, January 2023

Back Bay Books is an imprint of Little, Brown and Company, a division of Hachette Book Group, Inc. The Back Bay Books name and logo are trademarks of Hachette Book Group, Inc.

The publisher is not responsible for websites (or their content) that are not owned by the publisher.

The Hachette Speakers Bureau provides a wide range of authors for speaking events. To find out more, go to hachettespeakersbureau.com or email hachettespeakers@hbgusa.com.

Little, Brown and Company books may be purchased in bulk for business, educational, or promotional use. For information, please contact your local bookseller or the Hachette Book Group Special Markets Department at special.markets@hbgusa.com.

ISBN 9780316267656 (hardcover) / 9780316412834 (signed edition) / 9780316267755 (paperback)
LCCN 2021941531

Printing 1, 2022

LSC-C

Printed in the United States of America

To Peter

*I*f you are in Manhattan traveling downtown in a car on Fifth Avenue or Seventh Avenue and you want to turn onto Tenth Street, you have to turn left. It's a one-way street, west to east. Left on Tenth is my way home. I was left on Tenth when my husband died, and after that, life took many left turns, some perilous, some wondrous. This book is about all of them.

part one

Left

I knew my husband was dying in June. He'd been living with a terminal diagnosis for six years but suddenly his cancer turned aggressive.

The last time we saw the oncologist, he sent us home with a DNR (do not resuscitate) order and told me to put it on the refrigerator. "That's where they look," he said. He meant the EMTs.

I wanted Jerry to die at home. He wanted that too, but we didn't discuss it much. I was passionate about it, thought of it as a gift I could give him, to die in his own bed. The bedroom is sunny and the walls are painted a minty green. On days when he felt good enough, I figured, my husband, who was a writer too, could sit at his desk and write. If he needed to nap, which he did now almost all the time, he could nap on the couch where he always liked to nap.

We loved living on Tenth Street, a shady, pretty block in Greenwich Village. I couldn't bear to put him through his final exit somewhere else that was clearly only a place to die.

We redid our wills and updated our health-care proxies.

I began to rehearse being alone. I'd go to coffee with a friend or to some event and on the way home, I'd tell myself, *Imagine you are coming home and Jerry isn't there. He isn't there to share, to listen, to rant, to laugh, to comfort.*

Preparing for some unknown, for life without him, I also noticed that I needed to feel alive. I needed to walk fast on the street, get out, engage with friends. Dying was not where I wanted to be. I don't mean I didn't want to be with Jerry, but I felt, almost in a primal way, the need to feel alive. So there was a war going on inside—the need to be with Jerry, with his dying, and the need to be separate, an almost how-alive-can-I-feel.

I had met Jerry in my early thirties when I was finding my voice as a writer. My book *How to Eat Like a Child* came out the first year we were together. I remember hearing him in the next room laughing as he read it.

Jerry, a playwright and screenwriter, was in New York City doing the musical *Ballroom,* based on his television movie *The Queen of the Stardust Ballroom.* We fell for each other head-spinningly fast when a mutual friend brought him by my apartment. I felt I'd been looking for Jerry my whole life and he felt the same. He had a cropped beard and great hair, golden brown. His brown eyes were soulful, and his voice was smooth, a beautiful tenor. Arguments and difficulties over the years—the kind that all relationships have in their own specific ways—really only deepened our bond. We knew that we belonged together and the fact that we'd found each other was the luckiest thing.

Before Jerry, I wasn't someone who knew much about love. I was raised in Beverly Hills, the daughter of screenwriters. My parents were a team. They wrote films you might see now on Turner Classic Movies: *Desk Set* with Katharine Hepburn and Spencer Tracy, *Daddy Long Legs* with Fred Astaire and Leslie Caron, *No*

Business like Show Business, in which Marilyn Monroe sang, "We're having a heat wave." I'd been raised with expectations—all four sisters were expected to be writers—but my mother was cold to me and a drinker. She died in her fifties of cirrhosis. My dad was more loving but troubled and needy, a manic-depressive as well as a drinker.

Jerry was completely on my side. I'd never experienced that. I hadn't believed it was possible. He truly loved me and nurtured my talent. He guided me as I tried to master variations of the impossible: first my humor books, then essays, then screenplays, then novels. I could never have found my way without him.

Writers are writers first. Before anything else. It's a calling. Jerry and I both knew that and honored that in each other. I was wildly attracted to him and loved talking to him. He had a phenomenal understanding of human nature. He observed things I didn't, and I observed things he didn't, and talking with him about what people did and why was endlessly interesting.

Now he wasn't going to be here to love me or to talk to me. To have conversations with me about everything. Stuff. What was on his mind. What happened on the street. Why something made him or me happy or drove one of us crazy. He wouldn't be here to hang out musing about nothing while eating chocolate chip cake. To discuss all my writing problems or all of his. What a character should do, what another might be feeling, where to go from here. Jerry knew drama, could write it and teach it. He taught me.

He was raised in the Bronx in a big, extended shtetl Jewish world full of aunts, uncles, cousins, and vulgarity. Lively, yet full of phenomenal ignorance. Jerry had musical gifts. At a very young age, he could play any tune by ear on the piano. "He can play, why give him lessons?" his parents said. His grandparents made gin in the bathtub. His father sold costume jewelry. The little money they had, they gambled. His dad broke Jerry's piggy bank and stole his pennies. There were very few books in their apartment. It was a great world to write about, and Jerry did, but there was no one at home to nourish a writer's dreams.

Jerry was eccentric. We took tap-dancing lessons. Loved theater. Agreed on most things, liked to go to foreign places and do nothing much more than walk around and sit in cafés. Confiding in him was always comforting.

He was my true home. My first safe place.

At some point in September, Jerry was less able to walk around the corner, too dizzy to do the simple things like put Honey's bowl of water on the floor. Honey was our beloved little white Havanese dog. I talked to our internist and activated hospice care. We were assigned a social worker, a nurse, and a spiritual counselor. The only worship in our house was writing, but given that Jerry was dying and I was losing my soul mate of thirty-seven years, maybe one of us might want some spiritual help.

My recall is cloudy because I was anxious all the time, but I believe that, at the first intake session for home hospice care, I was told that if Jerry fell—and he already had once—I should call 911, but when the EMTs arrived, I could show them the DNR and health-care proxy. These gave me the right to refuse medical treatment for him. I should ask them only to lift him and put him back in bed.

I know I was given that instruction at least twice and maybe more by both a hospice person on the phone and a member of the team assigned to us.

Jerry was still able to walk if I held on to him, so after the first visit from the hospice nurse, we went to Pain Quotidien on a nearby corner, and while eating something like avocado toast, Jerry said, "Hospice. I don't know. I guess I feel okay about it. I don't feel anything."

"Sometimes it takes a while for you to know what you feel," I said.

That afternoon I came home to find Lauren, our sweet dog walker, and Jerry sobbing.

"What is it?" I asked as Lauren scooted by me out the door.

Lauren said she'd asked Jerry how he was, and he said, "I'm in hospice," and he broke down, and she broke down.

I almost started to laugh. This was so Jerry, to realize he was upset in an encounter with Lauren. But it wasn't funny. It wasn't funny at all.

I just stood there. I didn't put my arms around him. I don't know why. I just stood there.

This failure, this—well, really, this moment of abandonment— has plagued me, kept me up nights, made me feel that in spite of everything I tried to do for Jerry, I didn't succeed. I don't know why I failed him there. Was it my own fear and sadness about his death? Was I scared? Was it being unprepared for that moment, although I had no preparation for any of these moments? Why didn't I embrace him? Am I a cold person? Is being cold a safer place?

My husband's prostate cancer had spread to his bones. If I wrapped him in my arms, I risked hurting him, but every night when we fell asleep, he laced his fingers through mine. He didn't talk much about actually dying, and maybe this was my fault, because afterward it felt like everything was my fault. Maybe I avoided it, I don't know. Once we told each other that we were glad we'd spent our lives together. And Jerry said he wasn't frightened.

But I knew how much he missed me when I was out or at my

desk writing. "I need you near," he said, not in a demanding way, more with a certain amount of surprise.

He said the only thing he worried about was my being alone.

Jerry's last meal was Sunday, October 18, 2015. Zabar's tuna salad on a bagel. He sat at the kitchen table. We didn't know it was his last meal. We didn't know he would wake up Monday without an appetite, our first sign that his body was crashing. Zabar's, the wonderful market on the Upper West Side, makes great tuna salad, maybe the greatest. I guess it's not a bad last meal. A friend, knowing Jerry loved it, had dropped off some. I could get side-tracked detailing all the kindnesses friends as well as people we barely knew in our building showed us, leaving soup, homemade scones, and pasta.

Monday morning he got up, started shaking, and got back in bed. By Wednesday he was completely bedridden and foggy, and I was crying. I cried in a cab on the way to get a blow-dry. Do I need to explain why I was getting a blow-dry? I can't, except to say it's an addiction and I did not leave Jerry alone. These cell phones mean you cry and carry on in the most public spaces. I sobbed hysterically up Eighth Avenue while on the phone with my friend Lisa.

That afternoon while Jerry slept, I decided it was a good idea to pay his bills, something I'd never done. Insanity. I couldn't keep anything straight. (We had separate accounts and paid for different things, although both our names were on all accounts in case something happened to one of us. Which, now, something had.) I went into the bedroom and asked him for his ATM code. He reeled off his credit card number. I kept saying, "No, you know, the ATM where you go to a bank to get cash." He kept giving me the same twelve numbers. I wondered whether I'd ever seen anyone punch twelve numbers into the ATM. I started crying again. I left the room unable to believe I'd bothered him about an ATM code, feeling like a hateful person, then came back and apologized. He didn't know what I was talking about, didn't even remember. I clasped his hands. "Please forgive me for everything I have ever done to you."

"Everything?" he said.

The next time he tried to go to the bathroom, he managed to get only to the edge of the bed, where he collapsed, somehow on his back with his feet on the floor. He was drugged and not exactly uncomfortable, and being nearly dysfunctional myself, I was wondering if he could stay that way for a while—maybe until the night nurse showed up—when the buzzer rang, and it was Lisa.

Lisa was looking as she always does, simple and chic in jeans, a white T-shirt, and a blazer, her thick shoulder-length wavy gray hair in a lovely tumble. No makeup. Never makeup. She is a friend who's like a sister. Our backgrounds are similar. She is one of three sisters; I'm one of four. We're both middle children, which means we are always hoping/imagining we can make other people get along. She is immensely empathetic. We both had behind-the-scenes show-business childhoods and powerful mothers who fought for a place in a man's world. Hers produced films, mine wrote them.

Lisa suggested we use a chair to get Jerry's feet off the floor; then his feet would be level with his back. So we did that, and right after I went down to the doorman and managed to catch the building staff before they left for the day. They came in and, two on each side, lifted Jerry back into the bed. Jerry woke up then and brightened at the sight of Lisa. She sat on the bed with him, holding his hand, talking and laughing for an hour. They talked about our wedding, which Lisa was at, thirty-three years ago. They talked about *Hamilton,* the last play Jerry saw before becoming homebound.

"I'm so glad Lisa is here," he said.

Several times that day I had called my internist crying, and she decided to come down at five thirty to evaluate Jerry.

I left the room while she examined him. Shortly after, she told Lisa and me that she had detected pneumonia in one of his lungs. It came as a total shock. He and Lisa had just had a wonderful conversation. How could he have pneumonia? The next forty-eight hours, she said, would be critical. She ordered oxygen. His fogginess could be because his oxygen level was low.

At eight o'clock, the night nurse showed up, our first round-the-clock aide, and Lisa left. We live in a duplex and I asked the nurse to make herself comfortable downstairs and I would let her know if I needed her. I hung out with Jerry, stroking his head while he dozed on the bed, then I went into my office to visit my novel. Tinkering with my writing was always comforting.

I don't know how I suddenly realized he had gotten out of bed and was careening toward the bathroom. I shouted for the nurse. She came upstairs, and we caught him as he fell, breaking his fall but unable to stop it. He was on the floor. It was ten at night. As I had been instructed, I called 911.

I told them that my husband had fallen. He was on the floor. I'm pretty certain I said that the hospice had said to call them and get them to put him back in bed. Then I phoned Joel, one of our close friends, and asked him to come over. Jerry, meanwhile, seemed to be sleeping on the floor; he was snoring, and the nurse's aide and I were waiting. I called 911 again after a half hour, or what seemed like a half hour, and suddenly the EMTs were pounding on the door.

You can enter our duplex on the first or second floor. They came in on the first and Jerry was in the bedroom on the second. They charged up the stairs, angry at me because they couldn't figure out which apartment they were going to. I said, "How can you yell at me when my husband is on the floor?" The next thing I knew there were five EMTs in my apartment. It was startling. Later, Joel told me a few of them were paramedics. They were checking on Jerry, giving him oxygen.

I said, "I just want you to lift my husband and put him back in bed." I showed them the DNR and health-care proxy.

They said no, that Jerry was now under the jurisdiction of the fire department and he was going to the hospital. I protested. I waved the forms. I had asked my lawyer to make sure we were covered every which way. I was staring at the health-care proxy, paralyzed by the legal language, when Joel located the paragraph that clearly stated that I had the right to refuse medical care.

Meanwhile, Jerry was still on the floor.

"Well," one said, "in this case, we will take him to the hospital and you can show them the documents and bring him right back home again."

"That makes no sense," I said.

"Which hospital do you want to go to?"

I got my doctor on the phone to try and stop them. They refused to talk to her. She's not in charge, they told me. Now the person in charge is the fire department doctor. "Can he talk to my doctor?"

No, they said.

Around that time I realized there were two policemen in the apartment. Two cops just standing there. Five EMTs and two policemen. It sort of flitted through my brain that this was not a proper allocation of resources. They surely had something better to do in New York City.

Now the hospice nurse showed up. I got mad at her. "Why did you tell me to call 911 to put him back in bed?" She started arguing with the EMTs. I think she might have said to me, "Sometimes this happens."

My doctor on the phone suggested sending Jerry to Sloan Kettering because it had his records. I remembered that it had taken a while for Jerry to get admitted to Sloan in June. The patients on gurneys waiting to be treated or admitted in the emergency department stretched nearly to the outside door. The nurse suggested the hospice center at Bellevue. She called. They have a bed, she said. Jerry was still on the floor.

I started to cry. I swear I don't know if I was crying because I was so upset and so frustrated and so helpless and so sad or because I knew instinctively it was the only move left. I just started bawling and wailing. "I have spent months trying to keep my husband at home, doing everything I was supposed to, getting all the documents, everything so he could die here in his home with me, in his bed, and now you're telling me that he can't."

They got nicer.

I wonder about that. I wonder if they needed to bully me to tears, but they definitely got nicer. One said I had a sweet dog— this from the first EMT, the one who had been really mean. I realized that Honey had shrunk into a ball in a corner. Another noticed a series of photos of Jerry and me tap dancing together and complimented them. The woman, who I guess was the chief paramedic, said she would talk to the fire department doctor. It was up to him. In the meantime, they were going through all of Jerry's meds, asking me questions I couldn't answer. My brain was fried.

My husband was still on the floor and I wasn't even with him.

I was across the room, then I was in another room where the medical files were. I feel awful about that.

Finally they put me on the phone with the fire department doctor. He couldn't have been nicer. "Of course we would never interfere with your plans," he said, or words to that effect. "Of course we'll put him back in bed."

So they did. They all lifted him up and put him back in the bed. He snored loudly in what I assumed was a drugged sleep. I hope he slept through all of this, but I don't know.

The woman paramedic told me his vitals were weak. She said, "If anything happens later, please feel free to call us." I thought she was insane. It seemed to me that the other EMTs looked horrified, or maybe I imagined that. The two policemen who had stood there for forty minutes shook my hand and left.

All the EMTs left, the hospice nurse left, my friend Joel left.

I was worried that my husband might lurch out of bed again. I asked the nurse's aide to sit on the bedroom couch. I went downstairs to sleep. This was the first night I didn't sleep with Jerry. I couldn't sleep with the nurse staring at me. I think it was eleven thirty or so, I'm not sure. I called a friend in LA and told him the whole story about the EMTs. I called Jon, my wise and empathetic close doctor friend, and told him the whole story. Then I went to sleep on the couch in Jerry's office.

Sometime after three a.m., I woke up bone-tired. I lay there for a few minutes unable to move, then went upstairs. The nurse's aide appeared to be napping on the bedroom couch. Jerry wasn't breathing.

"I think he's dead," I said.

It seems so weird I said that just like that. Like I'd been beaten into bluntness.

The aide was shocked. She said she'd just been up with him and had fixed him up and straightened the bed, which had been wet and sweaty.

As we both stared at Jerry, he gasped. And that was it. He was gone.

I called Joel again, and my brother-in-law Nick, and my internist. They all came over. While I lay on the bed next to Jerry and they all sat around, we chatted about random things. Even though it was startlingly clear that he was gone, that the body was only a shell, it was comforting to lie on the bed next to Jerry. I told them about the EMTs.

A hospice nurse came by to certify Jerry's death: October 22, 2015, at 3:45 a.m. I told him about the EMTs.

Over the next weeks, to all my friends and family who took incredible care of me, I told the story about the EMTs. I told anyone who would listen.

$\mathcal{W}$hat I remember about the days after was how alien it was. With Jerry gone, I was dislocated, living in an unknown land. Traumatized by the events of his last night and tired from having been up nearly all that night, I couldn't recover. I was exhausted to the point of dizziness and at the same time charged on adrenaline. The apartment was full of friends and relatives. I remember coming downstairs from a failed nap and seeing a crowd in the living room, all of them chatting like it was a party. I felt as if I'd walked into the wrong house.

My dear friend Heather, who lives in Brooklyn, showed up at the door with her roller bag, moved in, and began organizing. I didn't ask her, it wasn't planned; she knew what I needed. She ordered food, ordered me to take naps, arranged everything. It was a phenomenal kindness. My sister Amy, who flew in from California, was helpful too, protective and concerned, and so was my sister Hallie, arriving later from Milton, Massachusetts. There were four of us sisters originally—Nora, the oldest, who is gone now, then me, Hallie, and Amy, who is the youngest. We were/are all writers.

In spite of knowing Jerry's death was coming, I had no idea what his memorial should be. But it quickly took shape in my mind. Jerry began as a playwright, and the closest thing to a synagogue or a church in our life was a theater, so I e-mailed someone I knew who was producing a play off-Broadway and arranged to hold the memorial at a small Greenwich Village theater the next Monday afternoon. Jerry had told me that he wanted his students to speak. There were four lovely, brilliant screenwriters whom he had nurtured and who'd remained close to him. Susannah, Phil, Alex, and Brian. I asked them and they agreed. I asked our very good friend Bob who had also edited Jerry's novel to speak. It's weird, planning a memorial. I've been to ones where they say anyone can speak, but I didn't think of Jerry's that way. I wanted it to have shape. A few people asked me if they could speak. I told them no. It sounds awful, but Jerry had never said anything about wanting those people to speak. I had strong feelings about how he would want to be remembered. I knew Jerry wanted to be known as a writer and a teacher. He had been heartbroken that his most recent play wasn't getting produced. We'd had a reading of it about six months before he died, and it was one of his happiest days. In addition to the speakers, I asked some actors who were our friends to read short bits of his play and his autobiographical novel.

I was happy with the service. It brought Jerry to life.

I never cried again. After sobbing my way through the EMTs, I was numb.

I was also seventy-one years old.

I had spent the past ten years dealing with death, which is I guess what happens when you reach a certain age.

My beloved sister Nora was sick for six years before she died in 2012. And her illness had been a six-year secret, an overwhelmingly difficult secret to keep. Secrets can eat you up. At least, that is true for me. Concealing something that big made every time I said I was fine a lie. My husband had been sick for ten years.

And it was possible I was sick.

My sister had had myelodysplastic syndrome, a disease of the bone marrow. Your marrow produces your body's blood supply. Myelodysplastic syndrome leads almost inevitably to fierce acute myelogenous leukemia (AML). Because AML can run in families and because the blood work done at one of my annual checkups showed that my red blood cells were getting larger—something that could mean nothing—my internist had sent me to an oncologist for a bone marrow biopsy in 2008.

This is not anyone's favorite test. They stick a needle in your hip bone, suck out stuff from your marrow, and test it. The results were that I didn't have myelodysplastic syndrome, although I had signs that I could get it. The doctor said that didn't mean I *would* get it.

Living through my sister's treatment, worrying about her, worrying about me, panicked about myself, guilty that I was worrying more about myself than her, plus worrying about Jerry and going through his treatment was a lot. I'd been living in a continual state of high anxiety.

Nora's doctors told her, after several years keeping her stabilized, that they couldn't do that forever and that she could have a bone marrow transplant, the only thing that might cure her. They discovered that she and I were a bone marrow match.

For what felt like an eternity but was maybe only six months, I waited for her and her doctors to decide what to do about it.

A bone marrow transplant, wiping out the sick marrow and transfusing in healthy marrow, is the only way to cure myelodys-plastic syndrome or AML. It often doesn't work. The body tries to reject the new marrow in all sorts of awful ways, a condition called graft-versus-host disease. Symptoms are terrible rashes, fevers, migraines, pneumonia, stomach problems, and heart problems, to name a few. But the transplant is more likely to succeed if you have a perfect match.

I was worried—no, *terrified*—about anyone messing with my bone marrow. And I didn't think the doctors were concerned about me, because they were Nora's doctors. Also, she was a national treasure—a writer and director, reinventor of the romantic comedy, admired by women everywhere. I was just, well, me. Or, as one of my doctors put it ominously, quoting the English saying, "the heir and the spare."

My worries ran wild. I imagined that I could save my sister but in doing so derange my own marrow and kill myself. Or I could attempt to save my sister, fail, and derange my own marrow—in this version, both of us would die. Or I could do nothing and still we would both die. Any of these scenarios seemed entirely plausible.

When Nora's myelodysplastic syndrome morphed into leukemia, I was with her every day in the hospital that last month. Watching her die was, in addition to the sadness, like staring my own death in the face.

A doctor who treated her and who did not know my situation said that dying of leukemia is awful. She was lucky, he said, she got pneumonia (which is known as "the old man's friend," because it can be an easier, gentler way to die than from your main illness).

I realized during this agony, during all this discussion of my bone marrow being used to save my sister, that I needed a great doctor. I needed my own advocate. My gynecologist said, "Take care of yourself, Delia."

Which is how Dr. Gail Roboz came into my life.

The oncologist who did my bone marrow biopsy told me about her. I had told him about my sister, and he said, "Dr. Roboz is brilliant. She is the top of the field in blood diseases." He said, "Maybe your sister should see her."

I thought, *I am going to see her.* I phoned and made an appointment.

Dr. Roboz was director of the leukemia program at Weill Cornell Medicine. My first thought when she walked into the small clinic room was *She could be my sister.* She was definitely from the same food group. Dark hair, brown eyes, slender, Jewish. Like somewhere, way back when, we could be related. Which was instantly comfortable and comforting.

And she was very alive. A force radiated off her. She was, I guessed, mid-forties, dressed beautifully under her white doctor coat, wearing high heels, and I believe there was some jewelry, like a bracelet or pearls. She looked like a girlfriend, and she had the warmth of a girlfriend, but she acted like a doctor. I mean, she had authority. She was absolutely in charge.

I poured my heart out. She looked at the results of my blood taken that day and at the results of my bone marrow biopsy and said, basically, *Right now, you're fine.* Having red blood cells grow larger didn't necessarily mean anything. She was relaxed about it. She agreed with the other doctor—I might get myelodysplastic syndrome, I might not. I asked if I could be her patient. She said yes. I should come back every six months and she would take some blood and see if anything was going on. She promised she wouldn't let anyone mess with my marrow in any way that was dangerous.

Ultimately, Nora's doctors decided it was too risky to use me to save her because my marrow might be diseased and that might make her sick again. Nora decided, in any event, she did not want a bone marrow transplant. There was no other perfect match for her in the system, which was unusual for Ashkenazi Jews, which we were. She read everything there was to read about bone marrow transplants and told me it was awful, grueling, the chemotherapy before and the entire subsequent process. She did not want to go through a long suffering. If you survived the transplant, your body might reject it. Also, you could just get leukemia all over again a few months later. Susan Sontag had had a bone marrow transplant, Nora told me, was tortured by it, and died soon after.

Also, Nora was over seventy. Because the process was grueling, doctors rarely attempted it on patients over seventy. But they sometimes did.

Of course I called Nora and told her about this fantastic doctor who looked like our sister, and at the end of Nora's life, she was under Dr. Roboz's care too.

After a while, I began to know more about Dr. Roboz. Not online things, like the fact that she had the highest academic standing in her Mount Sinai School of Medicine graduating class, but personal details, like that she loves opera. "It is," she said, "my drug of choice." She went to Hunter College High School, which is the public school for brilliant New York City kids. She married her first boyfriend, who also went there. New York City is Dr. Roboz's small town. Famous now in the field of blood diseases, she gives talks all over the world. She loves to mention her parents. She adores them. She will tell you, "Everything good about me is because of my parents."

Her parents are Holocaust survivors, both from Budapest, although they did not know each other there. Her mother, a young girl, evaded the Nazis by spending the war hiding in a basement coal-storage area. Her father lived in the Budapest ghetto. In 1956, during the Hungarian Revolution, when Russian tanks invaded Budapest, they escaped Hungary, separately but remarkably on exactly the same day. Her mother and grandmother trekked in the pitch-dark across fields full of land mines and eventually, with refugee assistance, made it to Vienna. There, her mother finished high school, and because of her intelligence, she was selected to study in the United States. Her father was plucked out of a refugee camp and sent to the U.S. Here they were fixed up with each other by Hungarian expats. They both became research scientists; her father, in his late eighties, still is.

Growing up with parents whose history was heroic and romantic as well as terrifying and traumatic, she was destined to save lives.

She always knew she would become a medical doctor. One day during her residency, she looked through the microscope at the cells of her first AML patient. A *coup de foudre*. She knew immediately that hematology/oncology was the specialty she wanted. "It has everything," she said of this complex, complicated field.

By the time Jerry died, I had been seeing Dr. Roboz for five years, and my blood work was consistently normal. As I recall, the last time I saw her before he died, she told me that my blood was the most boring blood she'd seen that day.

December 2015—one and a half months after Jerry's death

A friend told me this story.

She was on the beach with her ninety-year-old granny, her sister, her sister's husband, and their new large bouncy rescue dog, part Lab, part something else. They were all standing there talking. The dog suddenly charged and knocked the granny down.

To me, this is the story of a widow. Even a dog knows who the widow is. The widow is the weakest member of the pack.

It must have radiated off me, the sense that I was fractured. That I had suffered a blow. Did I look sad? I'm sure. In almost every conversation, I felt as if I were disregarded or not heard. At the cheese counter at the market; discussing a leak in the wall. Even waiters suggested I might order something other than I did. "That's a lot of dairy," one said to me.

About six weeks after Jerry died, I got what I assumed was a condolence note. It was from the spouse of one of Jerry's friends. It was the meanest note I've ever received. Actually, I had never received even a slightly mean note. He was married to the man who'd asked to speak at Jerry's memorial and whom I had told no. The spouse said I was an awful person. That the memorial was awful. That I cared only about famous people. That when Jerry was sick, his husband had offered to give up a weekend in the country to kindly stay with Jerry, and still I hadn't let him speak.

I am absolutely not someone who cares only about famous people. I know a few. A few are friends. None of the speakers at Jerry's memorial were famous. I don't "value" fame. Most of my friends have careers connected to the arts, but... well, you see what's happening—the minute I read this letter, I had to defend myself to myself. If the spouse wrote this letter, the couple must have spent hours trashing me. I would quote the letter exactly, but after phoning a mutual friend and reading it to her—and she was suitably shocked—I ripped it up and threw it away.

I had thought if you were the widow, you could do whatever you wanted at the memorial. Jerry had a relative who'd come down the aisle at her husband's funeral waving her arms, calling his name, and wailing loudly. She threw herself on the coffin. And everyone just thought, *Okay, Lulu needed to do that.*

I went to the eye doctor. I told him my husband had died. He said, "Of what?" I told him: prostate cancer. He asked what kind of treatment Jerry had had. Radiation or surgery? I told him radiation. He said, "That's why he died."

While my eyes were dilating, I got angrier and angrier. I said, "How can you say that to me? Are you saying it's our fault, we chose the wrong treatment?" He said, "Why are you upset? You made a decision."

Obviously I never went to that doctor again, but there was guilt in me, and he went right for it. Did I guide Jerry properly? Suppose we'd done surgery instead of radiation?

I went a little mad going over this. Should I have pushed Jerry to have surgery? I knew he didn't want it. If there were six side effects to something, Jerry would get seven. Empty nights after his death were taken up reviewing our choices. I discussed it with my very close girlfriends Julia, Deena, and Jessie. And with my friend Jon, the doctor, who told me that he'd made the same choices for his father that Jerry and I had.

Everyone reassured me. It helped and it didn't. I suppose whatever I did, it had to feel wrong, since Jerry was dead.

One morning I came downstairs and on the floor between the dining-room table and the hall was a gigantic bug. Just sitting there. A water bug, I think, but it was awfully fat for a water bug. I am bug-phobic. I hadn't killed a bug since I met Jerry. During all our years together, thirty-seven, he killed them all. I took a box of stationery—the cards I was using to answer condolence notes—and I threw it. It landed on the bug.

I waited for the bug to walk out from under the box. Nothing happened.

I was too freaked out to pick up the box. For me, seeing a dead bug can be almost as bad as seeing a live one. And I felt bad for killing it.

Nevertheless, I stepped on the box, pressed hard, and twisted it around. I still didn't have the nerve to pick it up. Once Jerry and I had dropped a brick on a large mouse and we called someone braver to come over and pick up the brick. The mouse was flat, like a cartoon mouse. Its skin wasn't broken but it was as flat as a penny. It was one of our favorite marriage stories. A sort of "See how suited we are." Even this mini-trauma, this you-are-alone-with-large-bugs-for-the-rest-of-your-life, reminded me of happier times, times I would never have again.

Taking out the garbage, I bumped into Jonathan, who lives across the hall. "Are you bug-phobic?"

"Not particularly," he said.

He picked up the box and, with a tissue, disposed of the squashed bug.

I should say something about my building, which I love. It has a doorman and it's a co-op, but it's a modest place, mostly one- and two-bedroom apartments (some combinations now; we have one, a duplex). It was built in 1928 for working middle-class New Yorkers. When we moved in twelve years ago, there was a cottage-cheese ceiling in the lobby and two urns. They sat on top of columns about four feet tall. Each urn held an unappealing green plant. This meant that our lobby bore a slight resemblance to a funeral home.

In spite of the soaring prices of real estate, the spirit of Greenwich Village is alive and well here. Residents are a mixture of gay and straight. There were three births announced at my first annual board meeting, one to a lesbian couple, one to a gay male couple, and one to a man-and-woman couple. There are writers, social workers, professors, a composer, psychotherapists, some museum curators, some magazine editors, and many retired people, as well as a few lawyers and Wall Street types. One of my neighbors works at the Metropolitan Opera. Another is a designer. No one who wants glamour lives here. No stars, no snobs. Very unglamorously, garbage cans are placed in front of the elevators for anyone to use between 8:00 a.m. and 10:00 a.m. At any other time, you take your trash to the basement.

We had made some close friends here, but people don't intrude. The board president thanks me if I complain.

There are about twenty dogs in the building. They are all nice. Even the two standard poodles who leaped at me when the elevator doors opened (one has since died) were nice, just rambunctious. If you have a dog, you know that once you name it, you immediately start nicknaming it. I called these dogs Howdy Doody and Clarabelle. It's the kind of building where you might nickname someone else's dog.

I was grateful to be living here, especially now.

There were tons of things to deal with. Jerry's bank and credit card accounts had to be closed, the co-op appraised. I had to dispose of his medicines (which could not be flushed down the toilet because they'd contaminate the water supply) and all the vitamins and potions he'd ordered off the web. Jerry had been trying so hard to make himself feel better. I hadn't realized this. There were many, many herbal medicines. Jerry did all the online ordering; humongous boxes of paper towels were always arriving. I guess these potions were too. It was strange to discover something even as simple as that, simple but emotional. Something I didn't know. I hadn't paid enough attention. Then there was the will. Death stuff.

I wanted to dream about Jerry. I wanted him to turn up in a dream. Because in a dream, someone can actually seem alive. They can be absolutely real. A dream was the only way I could spend time with him. I was thinking about that a lot, hoping that by thinking, I could make it happen.

And I did. And it felt absolutely real, as some dreams can.

In the dream, Jerry said, "I want a divorce. I'm leaving you." I knew he meant it. Jerry could be tough—not often, but when he was, there was no changing his mind. I left the room and came back. I said, "Well, I know you want to divorce me, but we can talk, can't we? I mean, if I want, can I just come over and talk to you?"

"No," he said. He walked down a hall and disappeared.

I woke up stunned.

Was that Jerry? Was that an actual visitation?

He was so mean.

I don't think dead people talk to you in dreams. That's always been my belief. I don't think dead people talk to you at all. I'm not religious or spiritual. I wish there were life after death but I don't think there is life after death.

Is there some sort of spirit world? I'm embarrassed even to type that sentence.

Extremely agitated, I thought about the dream for days. I told myself, *This is my dream. I created it. And in it, Jerry is telling me he's gone. He's left me. He was clear about it. He is never going to be in my life again. Except in memories. Get used to it.*

I was really shocked by this dream. It was an awful dream.

I should say right here that strange things have happened to me. Things that don't make me think there is a God or that Jerry could actually show up in a dream, but there is stuff going on in this world that science cannot explain.

A short detour:

When Jerry and Nora first got sick, I despaired. *How will I get through this? I am going to lose the two people that I am closest to in this world.* That night I dreamed the premise of a novel: Three women and a lion in a bar in North Carolina. I woke up with the characters and the title, *The Lion Is In.* I sat down and started writing that day. I had never gotten an idea for anything that way, and it was the most fun novel I ever wrote. Writing it gave my brain refuge for a couple of years. It provided the calm, play, and peace that only writing can offer me. I would go into my office and shut everything out but this story. It sustained me through the first years of their illnesses.

I had never been to North Carolina. Don't know why that location turned up in my dream. I did minimal research—chatted with a few people who had lived there, picked a rural area in the north of the state that my close friend Deena recommended. I had met Deena through Jerry right after we moved to Los Angeles, and since then, I rarely made a move without consulting her. Years before, she had written a screenplay that took place in North Carolina. After I completed a first draft, my writer girl-friends said there was no way I could set a novel somewhere I hadn't been. I had to go to North Carolina, to that area north of Rocky Mount.

I flew down to Raleigh with my niece Anna, a student at NYU who was always game for adventure. We drove to Rocky Mount. Every morning we would wake up at the DoubleTree hotel, get in the car, pick a random destination in the GPS, and instruct it to "take back roads."

We drove wherever the GPS sent us.

Now, in the novel, the lion, who lives in the bar, doesn't have a tree, and the woman who loves the lion finds a lone tree in a field. The tree looks like it's been struck by lightning. All the foliage is sheared off. There is just the trunk and some branches with the ends chopped off. As she says, it's more a sculpture than a tree. The woman convinces some men to dig up the tree and bring it to the lion.

As Anna and I were driving along on the way to God knows where, we passed an empty field, and there in the center, all alone, unmistakably, was the tree. The exact tree. Exactly as I described it. I screamed. We stopped the car. How could this tree exist? How could I have found it?

We got out of the car, and as I stared dumbly across the road at the tree, a man driving by in a pickup asked if anything was wrong. He told us that it was his friend's oak tree, the same kind as in my book, and that the bark on the trunk was rubbed off because the goats over there—he pointed to some faraway goats—went over and rubbed themselves against it. In my novel, the lion doesn't know what to do with the tree and rubs himself against it.

The man drove off. Anna and I stood there awhile. I couldn't even process it.

Then I wanted to see the inside of someone's house so I could write a better version of Clayton. Clayton, in my story, owned three things: the lion, the bar, and a vintage Chevy Bel Air convertible. Anna and I had lunch in a Mexican restaurant, and on a bulletin board, we found a card from a woman advertising home-made sweet rolls. We called her up, went to her house, bought some sweet rolls, and chatted with her in the living room. Her husband came home; we chatted with him too, and when we left, we saw his car parked in front of the house. It was a vintage Chevy Bel Air convertible. Top down, with a knockout-orange interior just like Clayton's.

These two events—finding the tree and then the vintage Chevy Bel Air—were exceptionally strange. They were more than coincidence, more than synchronicity. I couldn't slot them, categorize them. I dreamed an idea for a novel in a place I'd never been, wrote it, filling in the story and details, and then by random chance—was it random?—I found the very specific things that I'd imagined.

I admit, it flitted through my brain that I had some sort of special psychic powers. I could not believe I did or in fact that there even was such a thing, but still...

The day after Christmas I flew to Wales to visit Jerry's and my closest friends, Richard and Julia, to welcome in the New Year in their eighteenth-century farmhouse and cook on their Aga stove, which I love to do.

Richard, a beyond charming Englishman, had fallen in love with Julia just about the time Jerry had fallen in love with me, and we all fell in love with one another. They were both living in Los Angeles then and I had moved there to be with Jerry. Richard was a producer and Julia was a journalist. Now she's a successful novelist. We have shared all of our growth spurts as adults, advised one another and cheered one another. Richard is wise, a fantastic person to consult on all major life decisions. Julia is tall, redheaded, wildly positive, and so much fun. Her upbringing could not be more different from mine. Her father was a British fighter pilot in World War II and she grew up on army bases in places like Cyprus and was ultimately schooled in a convent. She broke horses in Australia before becoming a reporter. Julia has talked me into many adventures: canoe trips, a horseback ride on a mare she assured me was menopausal but who bolted across the meadow.

When they moved to Wales, Jerry and I visited often, terrifying ourselves as we drove backward (which is how I think of driving in the UK, where left is right and right is left) down narrow twisting country roads bordered on each side with tall hedges to their little glen on the river Wye. Their farmhouse was a place of comfort. We would talk way into the night and then at breakfast pick up where we'd left off. We also began meeting all over the place: Paris, Rome, Majorca, Cinque Terre, where they hiked (and I took the train) from one small town to another. In Lisbon when it rained, we holed up in the empty hotel ballroom and Richard taught us bridge.

We have memories of the four of us together, so many happy memories. Traveling together cemented our bonds.

They had visited Jerry and me in East Hampton three months before he died. We laughed—we always laugh together—and felt enormous tenderness about this loss coming at us. "I'll meet you on the other side, my friend," Jerry said to Richard when he and Julia got in the car to go to the airport.

I had told Julia that I wanted to come to them after Jerry died. I wanted to be comforted just with them.

I smuggled some of Jerry's ashes in my suitcase, in a baggie tucked inside one of my green ballet flats.

In Wales, it rained nearly nonstop. The only day the sun peeked through, we took a squishy little path away from their house to a spot where there was a peaceful view across a creek through ancient pines to emerald-green hills. A stone Buddha stood watch over the creek. Julia read from Wallace Stegner's *Crossing to Safety,* a novel about lasting friendship between two couples.

We tossed Jerry's ashes to the wind.

At night during the winter I tended to hang out in Jerry's office, a small room off the living room, eating and watching TV. I sold an idea for an original screenplay about publishing, and my novel *Siracusa* was scheduled for publication in July. I was also collaborating with doctors to create films to teach empathy to doctors. So I had work. Which I was able to do. Writing is my safe place. I know who I am when I do it. It's always been solitary.

Except, of course, now when I got stuck, I couldn't figure out my next move by talking to Jerry.

Heather, who teaches journalism and design at the New School a couple of blocks away, often stopped by in the afternoons to keep me company. Heather, who had moved into my apartment and seen me through the days after Jerry's death, is a friend-daughter.

I don't have biological children. I couldn't have them, and, after discovering that, I tried medically, but not too hard. The treatment was so sad—not getting pregnant was like a little death every month. Having my own kids, being a mom, had never been something I dreamed about. I was jealous of my besties—Deena (in Los Angeles) and Julia (in Wales)—when they were pregnant, but I loved their daughters. I let it go. Then I noticed as I got older that there were perfectly wonderful young women who had either lost their mothers or, for various reasons, could not connect well with the mothers they had. There is more than one way to get what you need, and I have been able to mother this way. It's not mentoring, although it may involve that. These friendships just happened, and I sort of figured out what they were afterward. They're my friend-daughters: Heather, Natasha, Jill.

Natasha is Richard's daughter, Julia's stepdaughter. She was raised in Los Angeles, and I share her with them. Sometimes Natasha and I sign e-mails to each other "sister/mother/friend." I try to model myself on Jill, who climbed Mount Kilimanjaro and trekked through Dogon country in Mali, a world where ancient villages are embedded in cliffs. I advise Jill on many things, but since I try to model her bravery and adventurousness in my own relatively tame travels, she is as much a friend-mother as a friend-daughter. In fact, they all are. The mothering goes both ways.

Heather is, I think, scary-smart and examines ideas like "the future of journalism." We met about ten years ago when a producer and I optioned a piece she wrote about women who hung out in a vintage-clothing store in Brooklyn. Heather also wrote a compelling memoir of her twenties and thirties called *Reckless Years.*

She would work in Jerry's office, and we would meet in the kitchen now and then. One day when she was here, I couldn't find her and realized she had been in the bathroom for quite a while. She came out. Sat on the couch, pale as can be, and showed me what was in her hand. A pregnancy test. We both stared. We kept staring, then checked the instructions. Turned the stick this way and that. Yes, she was pregnant. She was not expecting to get pregnant. She had a longtime partner, Oliver. The year before, at age forty-four, she had had her eggs harvested, and after examining them under a microscope, the doctor had informed her there was no way she would ever get pregnant.

We sat silently on the couch. It was truly a thrilling moment. Heather, always the realist, said, "What are the odds this baby is okay? What are the odds the pregnancy will last?"

She took another test. Fortunately, two came in the pack. Yep, she was pregnant. Life could still hand out prizes.

I took the sun setting personally. When the sun went down, I often did too. One time I fell asleep at 6:45 p.m. and woke up the next morning at 5:30.

People always asked, "How are you?" Emphasis on the *are* so I knew it was a serious question. But I never had a clue how to answer it. How did I distill this sad/lonely mess of me into something simple? I couldn't articulate my grief. And to try seemed to cheapen Jerry's memory.

They were being kind and thoughtful, but I disliked it. I know I would have disliked it more if they hadn't asked and if they had acted as if I were the same person I'd always been.

See what was happening? I was starting to get angry. I think, actually, I am an angry person, sort of—maybe it's just the detritus of being the child of alcoholics, having been denied a safe childhood, I don't know, or maybe being a woman in this man's world could make any woman mad, but without the sweetness of Jerry to moderate me, I was definitely getting angry. Actually, so were all my friends. And they hadn't lost their husbands. (I realize I hate the word *widow*. It's sexless. I'm never using it again.) The presidential election, Hillary Clinton versus Donald Trump, was occupying all airwaves, terrifying me and my friends about the future.

I avoided larger gatherings like book parties or any sort of party. I'd discovered, after trying a few, that I felt lost. More than that, I was almost panicky, looking around the room, wondering whom I should try to talk to. Also I felt that wherever I was, it was the wrong place. I really should be someplace else. But where? There was a continual sense of dislocation that I couldn't correct. Oh, I still had my apartment, but, much as I loved it, it was Jerry who made it home. I was, in a sense, homeless. Feeling like a stray.

I was lucky in my loyal wonderful friends and that I loved my block, Tenth Street, which was friendly and alive with people at all hours. In spite of all the changes in Greenwich Village, with NYU gobbling up buildings, and some new towering condos deranging the landscape, it still has a village feel. An intimacy. The "action" outside was comforting, a reminder that life goes on. When I walked by the antique-jewelry store Fichera & Perkins, Ron Perkins would wave at me through the window. Jerry had bought me two rings there that I cherished. I would go in to visit and Ron would cheer me up, gifting me with a chocolate bar. Ms. Lee at the dry cleaner's gave me a hug. I knew I could always stop at Il Cantinori, sit at the bar alone, undisturbed, and have my favorite dinner, grilled calamari and sautéed spinach.

I couldn't believe it when I survived to daylight saving, March 13. It seemed like a real accomplishment.

I made my first decision to move on: I decided to shut down Jerry's landline.

That summer I wrote an op-ed for the *New York Times*.

Love and Hate on Hold with Verizon

I know it's not a good idea to hate anyone. I know from an article I read today that negative emotion is bad for my health. I would hate to have a heart attack because my internet isn't working.

But I absolutely hate Verizon.

I spent four hours on the phone with them on a recent Saturday morning. I know for sure I was disconnected three times. Once I didn't realize it and just hung around for twenty minutes expecting someone to come back on the line. One person promised me he wouldn't disappear and even said, "Have I yet?" I said no, and then he disappeared.

I was feeling crazy that I was getting so upset about this. My husband died last October. I blamed my hysteria on the loss of Jerry, not to mention the long summer of the presidential election and the madness of Trump. With all this agitation and my own loss, I am for sure anxious and despairing. Feeling on all counts helpless.

At some point during my day on the phone with Verizon, at least two hours in, I had to go through all their prompts again. I yelled at the prompts. Prompts are sinister, because after Verizon disconnects you, you have to call back and obey the rules to get to anyone again.

While endlessly on hold, I wrote checks. Isn't that old-fashioned—paying bills by check? But actually at the moment it's looking smart. No internet needed. I wrote a check to Verizon for $145.88.

This all began because I disconnected one of my two land-lines. I don't need two landlines now that I don't have Jerry. This is the only change I have tried to make in my entire life since my husband died, and it has obviously not gone well.

One of my friends (not a psychic) suggested that Jerry did not want me disconnecting his phone, but honestly, that doesn't sound like Jerry. His voice was on the answering service and I recorded it on my cell phone before asking for the disconnect. He had a great voice—I was madly in love with his voice—and the only place I can hear it now is on this recording. He says, "You have reached Delia Ephron and Jerome Kass, please leave a message."

In any event, when I asked for one landline to be disconnected, somehow the company also disconnected the DSL on the other landline.

I know it doesn't make any sense, but that's how it started. Now, for the last month, Verizon has randomly disconnected my internet and I spend hours on the phone trying to get it back.

I feel bad that I yelled and swore at people just trying to make a living. But you know what, then I didn't feel bad because it was 10 p.m. and I still didn't have an internet connection. I had to call again, and someone said there was no record of an order.

I really did scream. I scared my dog.

Then I started thinking about gun control. I wondered, If I had a gun in my house, would I shoot the telephone? Then, being so agitated, would I forget that there were still bullets in the whatever-you-call-it, chamber, and one of the adorable children who visit me would find the loaded gun? In other words, I started thinking about hate and rage and how important it is to keep guns out of the hands of Verizon users.

It took nearly a week to get my internet back, and it's still erratic. I spend a lot of time with my computer at coffee shops. As a self-employed writer, completely dependent on the internet, I thought maybe I should sue for loss of work, emotional distress, and ten lattes. Internet access should be free. It's how people apply for jobs, communicate, find out what to do if they get bee stings or worse.

Being able to afford it is a great advantage. Hillary Clinton should take a position on this: "unable to connect" will end with her presidency. And throw in an end to all the robocalls too.

It turns out many people hate Verizon. I got hundreds of comments as well as e-mails sent to me through my website, all these people detailing their traumas with that company as well as with other phone companies.

Verizon called *me*. A woman named Rosie took over my problem, gave me her direct line, and said I never had to use prompts again. She permanently fixed my phone and internet problem. I guess the only way to get Verizon's attention is to write a piece that the CEO ends up reading at breakfast.

There truly are two levels of care. Probably everywhere. Not that I ever doubted that.

In addition to relating their own Verizon horror stories, a few men e-mailed vague things like *If you are ever in Hartford, call me.* Another asked me to have drinks with him at the Carlyle. I hadn't realized this column was a birdcall.

Drinks at the Carlyle? I discussed this development with my girlfriends. It was agitating to think of meeting a new man. I was pretty sure from his e-mail that this man wasn't my type. Drinks at a fancy uptown hotel...lovely for someone, but not me. He mentioned he had several homes and gave me the locations. He led with his money. I googled him. Yes, there he was.

My friend Jessie suggested that I didn't need to fall in love, but I could have someone, a guy friend who was sort of a boyfriend.

I e-mailed the man back and told him that I wasn't sure I was ready to see someone new. I wanted to think about it. I would get back to him after Labor Day.

That would give me a couple of weeks to ponder. A new life. A new man? I thought maybe I would meet him, but the idea needed to sink in.

In spite of my writing to him that I needed a thinking period, he e-mailed (I began to think of it as *bombarded*) me almost daily, suggesting other places to meet, all fancy, people whom I could talk to who knew him, like someone from Goldman Sachs. Even his assistant wrote for him, inviting me to an event in Connecticut. Was that supposed to charm me? Heather guessed his wife had been dead eight days. It was two months. I googled it. God, you can google anything. I mean we know that, but you really can google anything. His wife looked like a nice woman. I wondered if he had bet a friend that he could get a date with me.

I went so fast from feeling flattered to feeling bullied.

My mother had given me heaps of ambition—something I am immensely grateful for—but no guidance on men. "Pick one hairdo and stick to it," she told me when I was about eight. "You're pretty enough for all normal purposes" was another one of her favorites. As for romance/men/love, that was the sum of it. It took some therapy, and many unloving boyfriends, for me to find my confidence. Somewhere buried in me was still that vulnerable single girl. That feeling of wanting to be wanted, that girl I was before I became the woman I am.

My sensibilities had been so rattled by Jerry's death, I could feel that young girl banging around inside me, waiting to take me down.

There is a rule I live by: People begin as they mean to continue. I have sworn by that rule ever since the messy single days of my thirties. It was helpful in rooting out bad boyfriends as well as people I shouldn't work with. I did not answer any of this man's e-mails and still they came. I had told him I'd get back to him in three weeks. Was he stalking me?

I blocked him. But then, as happens, one e-mail popped through anyway. I had gone to a movie alone and I turned on my phone after the credits ended. He'd written a fake diary entry as if he were me at about age eleven, saying how much I liked him.

It was creepy. I nearly had a panic attack. And there I was in an empty movie theater. Feeling unsafe.

That night I consulted my friend Bill, a psychiatrist and a member of a group I'm part of called The Empathy Project. TEP is a collaboration of doctors and filmmakers who create films that teach empathy to doctors. After listening to the tale, he said, "I don't think he's crazy. I think he's immature. Write him a one-sentence note, don't use his name. Just say, 'Don't write me again.'"

It worked.

Is this what dating is? Is this what it's like if you put yourself out there? No different than when I was young?

I started checking out older men on the street—I guess old men, actually. I mean, I was old, they're old, we're all old—and rejecting them as they passed by. *His shirt's untucked. His glasses are lopsided. His hair's a mess.* It was obnoxious and immature of me, but self-protective.

A round that time, my speakers' bureau, which booked me for engagements around the country, told me I had been invited to speak at a conference of Jungians the following spring in Houston. I remember this so clearly. I had never been asked to speak at any sort of psychoanalysts' convention. I said to myself, *What's a Jungian? Before I go there, I'd better meet one and find out.*

I also thought—I remember this clearly too—that there were only two kinds of men I could ever be interested in, writers and shrinks. Because they both have emotional curiosity. This is ridiculous, of course. Lots of other men have emotional curiosity, and probably many writers and shrinks don't. Nevertheless, that childish, immature, but hopeful thought passed through my brain.

*I*n late September, I tried and failed to leave the country.

When I was trying to print out my boarding pass the night before my trip, I got this message: *Your boarding pass can't be issued. Arrive at the airport three hours early to have your passport verified.* I phoned Delta. The wait time to speak to a representative was two hours. I didn't wait.

I called first thing the next morning. The wait time was two minutes. "Why couldn't I print out my boarding pass?" I asked.

"You were randomly selected," I was told.

I moved up my departure from Tenth Street, leaving for JFK four and a half hours before my flight. In addition to being concerned about problems checking in, I also knew that the UN was in session. This is always a big deal in Manhattan. When the UN is in session, travel by subway—that is one of the many rules New Yorkers love to know. It was traffic hell all the way. Traffic so bad it makes you question your entire existence— where you live, what you love, why you ever thought a vacation was a good idea. Although I was going to visit Richard and Julia and their clan, whom I think of as my second family, and meet my goddaughter's baby, nevertheless... what had I been thinking?

I was positive I was going to miss the plane. I called Delta from the taxi and told them not to sell my seat. It was a points ticket. I am sure airlines regret points. I'm sure they regret everything about points. Because they are giving something away. Terms and conditions are not friendly. "Offers and benefits are subject to change without notice."

When I finally got to the airport, I told the agent I didn't have my boarding pass because I'd been "randomly selected." It didn't appear from his expression that he'd ever heard of such a thing.

He looked at my passport. "You can't fly to France," he said. "Your passport expires in less than three months."

"But I'm only going for five days."

"That's the rule. If it makes you feel any better, it happens to people every day."

"So the expiration date is meaningless?"

"Yes."

So I wasn't randomly selected. I was actually rejected.

I called Lauren, who was dog-sitting Honey, and told her she could go home. I texted Richard and Julia that I wasn't coming.

I couldn't bear to get back on the jammed-up highway. I took the air train, then the subway, which was pretty great, actually. It let me off at West Fourth Street. I had to drag my suitcase up several flights. Sometimes I want to scream at New York City, but then I just walk the ten blocks home.

Honey was happy to see me, leaping, licking, and emitting those yelps that sound like happy weeping. She'd dolefully watched me pack. She'd seen me leave. She thought I'd actually been somewhere. There is nothing like being welcomed by your dog. The sound of her paws racketing up the stairs the second the door opens. I ran her through her tricks: *Sit. Stay. Honey, come.* I gave her treats for each accomplishment.

Fortunately, back-to-back episodes of *Project Runway* were on and I didn't even mind that the commercials were longer than the show. I had a sandwich in my purse for the flight. I watched TV and ate it.

There we were, me and Honey. It wasn't France, but it was somehow fine.

October 22, 2016—the one-year anniversary of Jerry's death

I have now lived through Jerry's birthday, my birthday, our anniversary, and all the holidays without him. I've started to forget Jerry frail and sick but remember him more now as he was in health—a man with energy and joy. I like that better. Every day there are things I wish I could share with him. I have been able to write. I'm able to sleep. I love my friends. Honey gives me a dose of magic daily. I still get lost when the sun goes down. The silence in the apartment is loud. But I guess I'm okay.

I went down to the memorial for the victims of the 9/11 catastrophe, to those beautiful waterfall pools. I wanted to be someplace sacred.

part two

Peter

*T*hree days later, I received this e-mail through my website.

Your name: Peter Rutter MD
Your message:
Dear Delia—
Peter Rutter here. We know (knew) each other. Your big sister fixed us up when you were a Frosh at CT College, I at Columbia. My sympathies on the loss of your husband and sister. I am now a Psychiatrist/Jungian Psychoanalyst in the Bay area, and writing you because of several confluences: *Siracusa,* and your *Times* piece about disconnecting your late husband's phone, which closely matched my attempts to do so with my late wife's phone. They insisted I owed an early termination fee, even though she had the line for over 30 years; I did throw the "early termination" meme back at them, although currently the outcome is uncertain. *Siracusa* (loved the book): the last significant journey my wife and I made was to Sicily/Siracusa; we stayed at Domus Marie in Ortigia, which just about matches your cover photo. She was

also a Jungian Analyst, and died in March of lung cancer (not a smoker). I'm trying to heal up by hiking in and out of the Grand Canyon—done it twice in the past few months. I'm still working. We had 2 kids, now in their 30s, and a blessed granddaughter came along in September. If you have any interest in further conversation (clearly I do) email me or phone. [He included a number.] Be well, Peter

It was a nice note. Relaxed. Easy. Friendly. From a Jungian. I think, really, I was most stunned by that.

The amount of confluence was eerie. He came blessed by my sister. His last trip with his late wife had been to Siracusa, where my novel was set. It's a falling-down place in Sicily. How likely would that be? He loved my book. He knew the way to a writer's heart.

I had no memory of having a date with him.

I googled. There was his practice, in Marin County and San Francisco. But I could not find a photo of him. I mean, there were photos of many men with his name. All different varieties. I had no idea if one was him. But then I found books he'd written: *Sex in the Forbidden Zone* and *Sex, Power, and Boundaries.* I read some reviews. Good grief. How amazing. He was an expert in sexual harassment.

I immediately forwarded his e-mail to Jessie. I rarely made a move without consulting a girlfriend. Especially now, in this vulnerable time, my close girlfriends were my guardians. Jessie had been living close by while she was in New York, first writing the musical *Waitress,* then on a screenwriting and directing project. We had been having many coffees at our favorite café, Buvette, and I think I'd been weighing her down with my woes.

Jessie has a kind of spirituality; it's part of her wisdom. If she says, "You're going to be all right," it seems as if she must know that, that she's in touch with spirits from somewhere or other. She has a simple beauty like she's someone from the prairie, but she was raised in Southern California. She's full of charming contradictions: earthy and spiritual, compassionate and tough. More than anything, I believe, Jessie is someone everyone tells their secrets to. Especially about love. She is soulful and deeply trustworthy. So of course I sent Peter's e-mail to her.

Jessie wrote back: "I say this one is worth beginning a friendship with."

I waited a couple of days, God knows why.

Delia to Peter, Saturday, October 29:

> Hi Peter,
>
> Good to hear from you.
>
> I am so sorry about the death of your wife.
>
> Strange that you and your wife's last significant trip together was to Siracusa and you also battled Verizon over shutting down her phone. And your email handle is confluence. I once dreamed a premise for a novel and dreamed it without ever going to the place, ever, and when I went there, after writing the entire novel, I found things I wrote. Randomly. Like a particular tree even. That's not confluence, is it, nevertheless I went from believing nothing has any meaning to believing that everything does. Even though I'm often not sure what the meaning is.

Speaking of which, several weeks ago I accepted an invitation to speak at a Jungian conference in Texas and was thinking I'd better figure out what a Jungian is.

I am happy to say that as a result of having that piece in the *Times,* I have my own personal representative at Verizon and never ever have to do prompts again. Rosie is her name. Do you want her phone number?

Glad to hear you loved *Siracusa.* Thank you.

I'm embarrassed to say, I mean truly, that I have absolutely no memory of our date and I hope you don't either. Although being an analyst, you probably have better recall. Nora fixed us up? How did you know Nora?

Impressed you've been hiking the Grand Canyon. It seems so smart for a million reasons. I don't hike—unless you count across the Village to a bakery—but I respect it. I can see where, right now, where you are, it would test you, expand you, and remind you about how we're all passing through, a "tweak" to love it while you're here. A friend recently told me that Flagstaff has barely any lights at night and you can completely see the heavens. I was kind of craving that experience.

I am trying to figure out who I am exactly, this new whatever version. The writing stuff, assignments etc. keep coming, thank God.

I live in paradise, every day I walk outside and think, I can't believe I get to live here. And I have amazingly interesting and devoted friends and family, so . . . that's nice.

I noticed, googling, that you wrote *Sex in the Forbidden Zone* and *Sex, Power, and Boundaries.* That is you, I take it. How did that subject find its way to your heart?

Delia

From Peter to Delia the next day:

Hi Delia,

What a delight to wake up to your message, this dreary, rainy, darkening, always beautiful Northern California day. Your knowing that we do live in paradise resonates. Every line/sentence you wrote evokes much in response.

But because I have to rush out to see 3 generations of feminine lineage—daughter-in-law Alyson, granddaughter Idra born Sept. 2, and grandma Aileen from Texas (my son Naftali is showing his short film at the Savannah Film Festival)—I'll be brief (except for attachments below) just now, but more to come.

Books: Starting where you ended your message. Yes, I wrote those books, and in the first 20 pages of *SFZ* I describe how this problem arose in my heart. Thanks for asking in that particular way. The entire PDF of the book is attached. Since I've read more than one of yours, this one is on offer.

Confluence: It invokes so many levels and streams as you experienced in your-dream-to-waking-life and in the Texas invite. But it really started quite simply and geographically. Do you like puzzles? The photo below is me a year ago in a canoe about 50 miles upstream from a significant confluence. Care to offer a guess?

Nora: I had a summer job at *Newsweek* in 1962 as a nascent sportswriter, under Dick Schaap's mentorship. I fell in love with each and every one of the clip desk girls (they unanimously—and correctly—determined that I was too young for them). From that arose my meeting you, and I actually do remember much of it. We had several dates, including the evening your parents took us to see *Take Her, She's Mine* on Broadway.

I'm finding it terribly difficult to be brief so I will revert to that wonderful British sign-off:

Goodbye for now.

Peter

There were two attachments. His book and a photo. He was in a canoe. In still water. Some red-rock canyons behind. He looked just great.

How could I not remember him? We'd had *several* dates? He'd met my parents. He went to *Take Her, She's Mine* with them and me. My parents wrote that play. It was on Broadway my first year in college.

Peter told me much later that when he read "How did that subject find its way to your heart?" he said, *"Bashert."* He said it out loud.

He is not someone who talks to himself, he said. It simply slipped out.

Bashert is a Yiddish word, a word well known in Jewish culture. It means "destined soul mate."

I read the book's introduction. It was his story—about a patient who made him understand how the vulnerability of a female patient can play into a male doctor's fantasies and about his psychoanalytic mentor, who, he learned, was having sex with his female patients, and not only that, many of his colleagues knew. It was a gorgeous piece—personal, political, emotional, psychological. I can tell you that because later I reread it several times, but this first time, I sort of skimmed it. It was almost too much.

This was a substantive man.

I realized I knew someone who might know him.

I have a friend, Alice, who is a practicing psychologist living in the Bay Area. We went to high school together. She is my oldest friend. I called her.

"Oh my God, is he interested in you?" she said.

"I just got an e-mail from him. Off that Verizon piece months ago."

"I'll call you later. I'm in a car with four women on my way to our book group."

The next day she called. She'd met him, she knew his wife had died. She didn't really know him, but she did know a bit of his story—that he and his wife had been divorced for years before they got back together and married again.

I liked that. It made him more interesting. Wondering now why it made him more interesting, I guess I thought he wasn't conventional. And maybe he had more room for me in his heart.

Two days later, we exchanged five e-mails.

From Delia to Peter:

> Good grief. You went with me and my parents to *Take Her, She's Mine*. I don't even know where to begin with that.
>
> Several dates? The obvious question: Did you kiss me? A yes or no answer will be fine.
>
> You look happy in that canoe.
>
> Puzzles (Significant confluence): I can't even do a crossword, but I'm guessing it's AZ near Flagstaff. Near Red Rock Canyon. I went to camp near Flagstaff for many years when I was a kid.
>
> I read your opening. It's intense. Very intense. I appreciate how honest you were. My husband never backed away from a

feeling or reproached me for one, so I appreciate how fantastic that is. But it was hard to take in for me right now.

Have been nearly paralyzed by the latest election news. Could barely get out of bed Sunday morning. And now up in the middle of the night. Everyone I know is bananas. Have stopped watching TV or reading the paper—I really cannot take it. It feels as crazy as, well to overstate it, forgive me, but you know when you get really bad news, I mean with our spouses, and it's suddenly like being in a box and you can't escape. That's how I feel.

Hope you had a lovely time with your family. I got caught in the rain.

Delia

From Peter to Delia:

Delia—

I felt the tremor of your email in the middle of the night, and know the feeling of the box you can't escape. I feel I have one foot in and one out of that box. I completely share your anxiety about the election. I am driving to Reno this coming weekend to canvass and get out the vote for Hillary and Catherine Cortez Masto, who is in a very close race for Harry Reid's Senate seat. If she wins, she will be the first Latina US senator.

A yes or no on the kiss back then—No. [ ]

The canoe photo is the Colorado River near Moab, UT, at the beginning of Cataract Canyon, about 50 miles upstream from the confluence of the Green and Colorado Rivers, which together do their work carving Glen Canyon (now largely covered by Lake Powell) and Grand Canyon.

These are the easier answers; there is so much more to say about everything else in your/my messages.

Do you feel up to having a phone conversation? I'd like to whenever it might suit you. You have my number or send me your number and a good time to call.

Goodbye for now,

Peter

From Delia to Peter:

A phone call?

All I know about Colorado is Denver is there. Truly, I am a city girl. Important to know, important to believe.

As for tremors, you live in Northern California, so that was probably an earthquake and it's a good thing you're going to Reno unless it's some sort of appointment in Samara situation and the quake is there.

It's great that you are going to Reno. Really great.

Okay, seriously, I don't understand this connection, which clearly exists, I mean, I'm a little gobsmacked and I am scared, actually plain scared, and scared of missing Jerry more by talking to you. I don't mean it the way it sounds. I'm sure you know exactly what I mean and will miss your wife more by talking to me. There is some way I understand this going forward, the fierceness necessary, and yet there is something about death that makes me more interested in life than ever. Paradox is everything, but truly I can't believe I am emailing a stranger something this personal. So I am confused by all this.

Let me think about it overnight.

D.

From Peter to Delia:

> Delia—
>
> Of course: that is, to your thinking about it overnight, or whatever inner dimensionality you find you need.
>
> I think you got the meaning of my thus far unsaid, therefore empty-bracketed thoughts/feelings: [ ] They are plentiful.
>
> Yet there are a very few things for now that I do want to say:
>
> There is no one else, nor has there been since Virginia died, nor did I expect such.
>
> This will be nothing more or less than what our confluence alchemically creates.
>
> Although we are still strangers in some sense, despite our past either mythic or real connection, there seems to be some mutual recognition of the other as a potential close ally.
>
> Another recognition appears to be the perception that neither of us is prone to back away, as you so beautifully attributed to Jerry (I admire that in him), until there is a damn good reason to back away.
>
> And yes, I have already consulted Virginia, not that I really know how to do such a thing, but cried when I did it, knowing (in her gone-ness that will always be part of me) that she would wish me to go ahead and find out what this is.
>
> I believe our hearts will tell us how to do this.
>
> P

I would have been out of my mind not to talk to a man who wrote a note like that. "Potential close ally." How gorgeous was that? A yes or no on the kiss? "No." He had answered as I asked him to. That told me a lot. He listened to what I asked. He respected boundaries.

The thoughtfulness. Yes, I dissected every inch of his notes. We set a date for a call. I wrote him that I was going to buy boots.

Peter sent me a song, "Come in Stranger," by Ian and Sylvia. He wrote, "In addition to your boots, two minutes to help prep you for an upcoming conversation with your new stranger."

"Come in Stranger" is a wonderful folk song that dates us both: "Stay long enough so the one I love won't be a stranger to me." Then he sent me another: "You Were on My Mind." And then another as we heated up: "This Wheel's on Fire." He was courting me.

I was driving Jessie nuts by now. *Waitress* had opened; she was writing and preparing to direct another musical, *Alice by Heart*. Still, she found time to listen to me carry on about whether I could do this or couldn't do this, and all the while, of course, I was doing it. If you catch a wave and it's right, you are gone. The momentum was out of my hands.

Our first phone call was on Tuesday, November 1. I called Peter from my landline, sitting on a couch in Jerry's office. Why did I put myself there? I guess to make it as difficult as it could be for me. I was so anxious. I would hear his voice. Would he have a nice voice? He would be real now, not just an e-mail personality.

All I remember was wanting to get off the phone. His voice was just fine, not smooth like Jerry's, deeper, with a roughness to it. I don't remember what we said. Not one thing, except I said I had to get off fifteen minutes after we started talking. He was a bit surprised and asked if he could call me later, after his next patient. (I think now of all the shrinks and what could have been happening in those ten minutes between patients.) He pressed on that. I said okay. I talked to him an hour later in my office. Not for long.

I am someone who needs to adjust to everything. A few steps forward, a few back—that's me. That has always been me.

And one single thing about all this: We were both seventy-two and age meant nothing. We were getting as loopy, as obsessed with each other as anyone falling under the spell of romance.

We made a plan to speak on Friday, several days later. Peter sent another Ian and Sylvia, "Tomorrow Is a Long Time." I wrote back, "That song is deeply romantic." Peter wrote back, "As, you can't help but have noticed, am I, my dear."

Short e-mails were now flying back and forth, and Peter was going to drive to Nevada to canvass. We talked the four hours there and the four hours back. We talked about everything, God knows. I probably knew some of his life since we'd had several dates, one of which, Peter said, was at a Columbia football game. I had a dim memory of being at a Columbia football game, not of who I was with, but of snow falling. The brain is a strange thing. Yes, Peter said, there were snow flurries. Peter recalled our talking in the stairwell of the Algonquin Hotel. That was where my parents always stayed. He did not have any memory of their being difficult or alcoholics or anything about my chic mother with her short hair brushed back, her stylish suits, and her scotch old-fashioneds consumed one after another. He did not remember any tension between them, although they had a bitter angry marriage. All he remembered was he and I talked. But not about what.

Peter, I learned, was a New Yorker. He grew up on the Upper West Side at 102nd Street and Central Park West. Like me, he is Jewish with parents whose main allegiance was to left-wing politics. His parents divorced when he was five. When he was seven, he was on the park side of the street, playing with his friends, when he heard a scream and a crash. His mother and sister were lying in the street, hit by a car.

He never saw his mother again. She lingered in a hospital for a short while and then died. He wasn't taken to the funeral.

His sister survived. She had a broken arm and two broken legs. About two months after the accident, she came home. His father, not a kind man, moved back into the apartment. Peter and his sister were never allowed to mention their mother.

Many of us have tragedy—I certainly got scarred by the rage in my parents' house—but his was particularly severe and sudden. It obviously shaped him, explained why he ultimately decided not to be a sportswriter but instead go to medical school and become a psychiatrist. Two of my close friends lost their mothers suddenly and tragically when they were children. Jessie, whose mother died when she was three years old, calls these survivors members of the Dead Mothers Club. An exceptionally empathetic group, she says. That is true of Peter. He is truly understanding. His life, he felt, was saved by the Quaker camp in the Pennsylvania wilderness that he was sent to every summer and where he learned how nature could heal and provide peace. That's why he was hiking the Grand Canyon after his wife died.

He was interested in me. "Tell me more about that" is something Peter always says, said from the start. Like Jerry, he never reproached me for a feeling.

We talked about sexual harassment. I hadn't realized it wasn't even against the law until 1986 when the Supreme Court, in a unanimous decision, declared that sexual harassment fell under the Civil Rights Act of 1964. Before that, it wasn't a recognized offense. Peter had lived his beliefs. He had spent a decade testifying on behalf of abused women in court.

He believes everyone should be able to have psychotherapy, and he accepted both Medicare and Medicaid in his private practice. In the years when he was divorced, he worked in clinics in Napa County and Midtown Manhattan where many of his patients were

undocumented, homeless, or trying to kick street drugs. He'd
practiced in Boulder. His life had been a winding road, but it was
the journey of a healer.

Just generally, I love talking on the phone. Texting and e-mail,
which have mostly replaced it, have deprived me of endless conversations with friends. Peter and I were simply voices connecting,
spilling our thoughts. Getting to know each other. It was a fantastic
adventure.

Very late at night, Delia to Peter, nine days after receiving his first
e-mail, only a subject line:

> I MISS YOU.

Later than that, Peter to Delia:

> Likewise, sweet D.

We hadn't yet met.
We had a plan, though.
Peter would fly to New York to see me the following weekend.
In the meantime, my days were occupied with trading e-mails, my
nights with long phone calls. It was as if the universe had given us
a gift—to experience all the madness and thrill of falling in love
at a time in our lives when that was supposed to be over. It was
happening at the speed of light. Which is the way it had happened
only one other time in my life, when I met Jerry.

This was, I guess, the most clinching exchange. Because it was
about money. I knew I couldn't be with anyone who was cheap.

How could this man be cheap? But still, I had to know. I called it "a prayer," but truthfully, it was a test.

Delia to Peter:

> Darling Peter,
> Here is my prayer for today.
> That you tip easily and well.
> That you know other people work hard at things we don't want to do, and they should be rewarded for it.
> That, when you split a check, you never ask someone else at the table, "How much are you leaving?"
> That you pick up checks easily.
> That, when you split a check, you just split it down the middle.
> That you hand over your credit card without looking at the bill (except maybe in dive bars in foreign countries).
> That is a lot to ask, I know. And yet it is central.
> Your besotted but ever wary,
> Delia

To Delia from Peter later that day:

> Dear Besotted and Wary—
> I woke up just before your email came, checked, no message yet, drowsy in bed, missed you, missed your hand and more next to mine, wondered, Where is she?
> Comforted myself that I would hear any sec, and then your email came!
> I score a perfect 10 on everything—if not better. I especially

like leaving at least 20 percent even if the service was flawed; this is part of a server's wage of a generally thankless job. I am a proletarian to my bones and feel above no one. I never look at a restaurant check before I happily throw my card on top of it—when it comes back, I look only long enough to calculate the 20 or more percent. The one thing you left out asking: Yes, I calculate from the tax-included bottom line.

In Europe, always some euros on the table on top of what they automatically add to the check.

Who knew that these considerations between us would be what we need to know to close the deal?

But they should be.

Your (and I mean that deeply and powerfully) Peter

The day of the money prayer was also Election Day when Hillary Clinton lost in an Electoral College upset. I went to my brother-in-law's to watch the returns and got almost sick realizing it wasn't going her/our way. It was splintering, to feel so much joy personally and so much despair about our world.

The night before we met, Peter to Delia:

From our grief we have found each other.

We will do right by those who helped bring us here.

Precious one.

Hope you are sleeping peacefully and let this touch you deeply when you awake.

Delia, je t'adore.

From Peter, the Come In Stranger who is absolutely yours.

Our first in-person date was Saturday, November 12. Reading these e-mails, I can't believe all that transpired between us without a meeting. Looking back, we were already in love and possibly set up for catastrophe. The phone calls and e-mails were almost dreams, perfect versions of ourselves.

I worried about Peter coming into this apartment, which was still very much mine and Jerry's. Worried that it would be hard for him. That it would be hard for me too. Photos of Jerry and me together, framed posters of Jerry's work on the wall, his clothes in the closet. Peter, I had learned in one of our calls, was living in a new place, an apartment in Mill Valley. He and his wife had wanted to sell the house to give their children down payments for homes of their own. He moved out two weeks after her death.

With Linda, my beloved housekeeper of over twenty years, kindly bossing me around, I put Jerry's clothes in the basement box for Goodwill, cleared off his desk, moved his computer to a closet. Hardest to part with were his eyeglasses. They were sitting on my desk, to the left of my laptop and a little bit back. Very comforting to see them, a way of having him with me when I worked. Why did I toss them? I don't know. I was in a bit of a frenzy. I still regret it.

The day of our date, I had a blow-dry. I went to Bergdorf Goodman because I knew a makeup artist who worked there on Saturdays and she spruced me up. I wore...something...I think my black leather pants and my pretty black blouse. Boots, for sure. They give me confidence. We had a reservation at Cherche Midi, a charming downtown bistro. Jessie knew someone there and arranged the table. I called her multiple times to make sure we could get a table in a corner—it could be noisy there, and it would be good if we could hear each other. I was frantic, Jessie was patient. Peter and I could walk to Cherche Midi from my place. "What? You let him come to your apartment?" a friend said. I don't remember which friend. She had no idea how far these e-mails had taken us.

I took off my wedding ring.

Seeing him in person was almost deranging. He had dark, deep-set eyes, white hair, and a great quick smile. I loved his smile. Gorgeous laugh lines in his cheeks. He did not take his eyes off me—in my memory anyway—but fixed me with such a happy look. He was about five eight, perfect for my five three.

He brought me a rose and a little stone animal made by the Zuni people, a fetish, a souvenir of the Southwest, his spiritual home.

We went into the kitchen first and I didn't want him to sit in Jerry's breakfast chair. Not that I told Peter that. Nor did I say that Jerry was with us. There were definitely three in the room. I couldn't let Jerry go. The kitchen is narrow, so I was nervous because Peter was close. We moved to the living room.

Our conversation had almost no intimacy, but the atmosphere between us was charged. At dinner I was so tongue-tied, I asked him his favorite color. And then again noticing how happy he was just looking at me, I said, "We're not getting married this weekend."

We both started laughing. I think that's when things eased up, but as I said, I don't really remember. I do remember that we shared a raspberry soufflé, which is one of my favorite things. When we left the restaurant, Peter kissed me. Not lightly. A wonderful, serious kiss. On the corner of Houston and Bowery.

Now with his arm around me, holding me tight, we walked back to my apartment and made out on the living-room couch like teenagers. We had great chemistry. Sometime after midnight, he returned to his nearby hotel.

When I woke up the next morning, I was zonked. Physically and emotionally. And freaked out. We were supposed to meet at noon in Washington Square Park. *I can't do this,* I thought. *I can't start some new life with a stranger. I can't turn my life over, begin again. And then what? Then what? One of us dies?*

I called Jessie. I was close to hysterical. "I can't do this," I kept saying. "Maybe I just want sex." I think I might even have used the term *fuck buddy.* I had never in my life used that term. I am way too old for it. I have no idea how it even popped out of my mouth. I was panicked. "He has a backpack," I told her.

Now, he did have a backpack. A beat-up blue backpack that looked like it had been all over the world. He didn't take it to dinner. He was actually dressed beautifully, in a suit and a black overcoat. Until I mentioned his backpack to Jessie that morning on the phone, I hadn't even realized I'd noticed it.

"Every man in Northern California has a backpack," said Jessie. "Get over to the park."

I walked Honey over. The park on a fall Sunday was its usual, teeming with people of every age and variety, noisy with conversation, children, and dogs. That guy who wheeled his baby grand over every weekend (how did he do that?) was playing. I turned in circles and finally spotted Peter some distance away, at the fountain, looking around for me. I waved. He smiled but then read the anxiety on my face. I saw his welcoming smile wipe off.

We sat on a bench. And we talked. We really talked. With all that chaos around us, almost oblivious to it, we had a serious conversation. About what it meant to start something intense and meaningful at this age. To fall in love now, when death is right there in front of us. When we can reach out and touch it.

I told him a little bit about my medical situation—that I had abnormal cells in my bone marrow that were harmless right now and might remain so and that the doctor had been tracking me for seven years. I had mentioned this on the phone, but I brought it up once more. Neither of us should have to go through again what we'd both already gone through, Peter with his wife, me with Jerry. I said, "If I get sick, I give you total permission to leave me."

I didn't really mean that. It was almost a joke—I have a tendency to spin serious things that way.

Peter said, "I could never do that."

There it was, right there, our different natures: Me trying to amuse, trying charmingly to deflect fear; Peter dead serious. "I could never do that."

I was almost taken aback that he wouldn't joke with me. That he put a period on it. That was his character. *I could never do that.* I didn't totally understand it at that moment, but thinking back, as I have over these times, his constancy was evident.

Now spilling everything, I also told him that this was a lot. It was too intense for me to spend three days with him. I didn't want to feel "trapped." I made a big deal about that word. We needed to get to know each other. I needed to go a bit more slowly. He said, "Why don't we take today? Tomorrow I'll visit my friends in Brooklyn."

Peter, I was learning, always heard what I said and never tried to argue me out of a feeling. Of course, the minute I expressed my anxieties and he said it was fine, I relaxed. We took a long walk through the Village to the Morton Street Pier. Peter held Honey's leash. He was charming even my dog. We looked out at the water, watched tugboats chug upstream. Peter stood close behind me, his arms wrapped tight around my waist.

We stopped for pasta at a local Italian place he'd eaten at over the years whenever he had been in the city, then went back to my apartment and spent the rest of the day and night in bed.

From me to Peter the next afternoon, November 14:

> Peter,
> You must be on your way to the airport.
> Heather is in labor so I'm very excited.
> I didn't thank you, such a strange thing to say, but I didn't thank you for taking me out, for coming here, for being considerate and kind and exciting, for giving me room to breathe and taking my breath away, for your hands and your heart and all the rest of it.
> D.

From Peter to me:

D—

I miss you but feel so much gratitude for all that has happened between us in such a short time, so that fills me up even in the missing.

Please breathe well and don't be trapped.

Good-bye for now,

P

Heather and Oliver have a beautiful baby boy, Rowan. I am sort of a grandmother.

Creatively, my year has been good. My novel *Siracusa,* published in July, inched briefly onto the *New York Times* bestseller list, and at the end of the year it got lovely mentions in magazine wrap-ups.

Peter and I spent the next three months falling in love. I visited him for five days. A shockingly long time, but I told him, "If it gets difficult, I'll move into a hotel." It wasn't difficult. Peter went to his office every day to see patients. I stayed in his one-bedroom apartment, shaded with redwoods. I wrote in the morning. At lunch I took a steep dirt path to the street and then a ten-minute walk into Mill Valley—a town that feels like East Hampton crossed with Canada. I mean, it's a wealthy little village with expensive shops, but its visual is rustic. The café in the center of town made delicious clam chowder and excellent cappuccinos.

Peter took me to his favorite places: An hour north to Point Reyes to whale-watch. An hour south to Monterey, where we got caught in the most horrendous traffic jam. Traffic is bad here—can you cross the Bay Bridge before this hour or not, go south on the Golden Gate after that hour? Everyone debates it.

I visited with two close friends. Alice, my high-school pal who lived in Berkeley, drove over. Since she knew Peter—barely, but she did—and was a psychotherapist, so a colleague (at least I think these were the reasons), she felt that she could tell Peter he'd better be good to me. Seriously. I could not believe she said it, practically poking her finger in his chest. I did feel I could take care of myself. I took an Uber to have lunch in San Francisco with Meredith.

Meredith and I have had a long, intense friendship, even, unimaginably, a time when we didn't speak, which was repaired instantly when she called me the morning after Nora died. I remember sitting up in bed, numb; the phone rang, and it was Meredith. And bang, we were close friends again. I don't know why we stopped speaking. I can't even bear to think about it. She is from New Mexico—a desert-and-big-sky woman—and has a radiance, both grace and charm. And an infectious laugh. Men fall in love with her across rooms. Also, she has a steel-trap brain. She knows a phenomenal amount about medicine and is compassionate and wise about it. As a television producer as well as a newspaper and magazine editor, she has assigned and edited hundreds of medical and science pieces. She has also had several medical issues herself, so she understands the patient as well as the science. Medically, I have always trusted her advice more than anyone's. She misses New York City like crazy. Whether to move back is a continual debate. She comes east for a long stay every few months.

Now I might be coming west to her. She knows all the good bakeries in San Francisco. I had a fantastic slice of gingerbread. I love gingerbread. *This will work,* I was thinking. Oh, not exclusively. I mean, Northern California would work as a beautiful alternative to my New York City life. Friends assured me it would be good for me. I'd become "too" NYC.

Peter told me more about deciding to call me. It had been simmering, he said, since he read my Verizon piece where I mentioned the loss of my husband. He didn't actually decide during his second Grand Canyon trek, down to the bottom and up in one day. This hike—with his friend Jim—was so arduous that he couldn't think about anything except the next rock in his path and would they get out of the canyon before dark? But afterward, he said, his head was clear, and as he drove through the desert and then to Tucson, taking all back roads, loving the landscapes, he realized several things. He would try to contact me, he would retire in two years, and, if I didn't work out, after his retirement he would get a camper van and travel the Southwest.

I met Peter's son, Naftali, his wife, Alyson, and their baby, Idra. We had Chinese takeout in Peter's kitchen. Naftali was a filmmaker; Alyson, an actress and theater director, also taught acting. Alyson was exceptionally warm. She was a pretty redheaded Midwestern farm girl who loved New York City as much as I did. Naftali, tall and intense, liked to be in charge, as directors often do. I was nervous, they were curious. Before they left, Naftali asked me if I liked classical music. It was a test question. Peter loves classical music and opera. I don't dislike classical music, but except for an obvious Mozart concerto and a Vivaldi, I am an absolute ignoramus. I did not say, *No, I only know show tunes.* It's too pathetic—music and me. A great failing. "Not really," I told him, "but I'm open to it."

Peter's daughter, Melina, was a public-school teacher, an accomplished young woman who spoke many languages and taught drama to kids whose first language was Spanish. She wasn't ready to meet me. Which was fine. I wasn't really ready to meet her either. I hoped eventually we'd all be friends.

Somewhere in here we went to Los Angeles, where I lived for most of my adult life before moving back to New York. I had many friends there, including Jerry's screenwriting students who moved there and had careers. Bringing these young talented writers into my life—they were smart, funny, loyal, and warm—was one of the greatest gifts Jerry gave me. Introducing them to Peter was hard. I knew they would feel Jerry's absence the most, and with them, I would too. I remember Fia's reaction—Phil's seven-year-old daughter—the utter confusion on her face when I walked into the kitchen with Peter. Like, *Who is this?*

It would never be cozy the way it was. But it was okay.

Peter and Deena bonded over their love of baseball. Deena, a rabid Dodger fan, saw Sandy Koufax pitch a perfect game when she was twenty. There have been only a handful of perfect games ever pitched in all of baseball, Deena explained to me. Koufax got every single batter out in succession for nine innings. It was stunning and sealed her love permanently. She was Jerry's close friend first. When I moved to LA to live with him, there she was, and I needed the world's best girlfriend. Truthfully, I sort of stole her. At that time Deena and I were both budding screenwriters. Now we are both novelists. It was an instant bond. If I have any sort of problem—writing, business, personal—I call Deena. We are on the phone for an hour at least once a week discussing every single thing in our lives.

Everyone liked Peter, it seemed to me. How could they not? He was nice, he was perceptive, he was interested in other people, which, God knows, was a gift, and I was so happy.

I tried to push away my guilt. All my friends said, "Jerry would be so happy about this." Really, everyone assured me that Jerry could not have been happier. It was kind of them, for sure. I certainly would be happy if I had died and Jerry had found someone. But all this sex? Would he be happy about that? And I want to apologize for even mentioning sex. No one wants to hear about two seventy-two-year-olds getting it on. In a movie, I know, if you have two seventy-two-year-olds simply kissing, you want the camera far away, like across the street or out the window. But our attraction was an essential part of the magic.

I told my gynecologist I had met a man. She said many of her patients who'd lost their husbands found men they had close friendships with. I said, "It's not really like that. It's pretty intense."

My neighbor Mitch, who lives with Stephen—both of them are my close friends—asked only if Peter had good hygiene. I assured Mitch he did.

This replay of young love when I am old—heady, giddy, exhilarating—I was aware every second of what a gift it was. At the same time, there was something lurking...something, I learned from Peter, that Jungians call the shadow.

E-mail from me to Dr. Roboz a few weeks after meeting Peter:

> Hi Gail,
> Quite miraculously, I seem to be falling in love.
> (With a psychoanalyst. An amazing guy.)
> I told him that Nora and I were a genetic match and that I am tested every six months to see if I have her disease.
> Is that the accurate honest thing to say?
> I'm not sick and there is no predicting it, is there?
> But I have to be straight. I have to tell the truth.
> I ask this with great trepidation, I realize.
> Delia

From Dr. Roboz to me:

> Wonderful news, congrats. The fact that you and Nora were "matched" for transplant doesn't mean that you are

genetically predisposed to get MDS, which is rare in families. So, you don't need to imply to him that you will definitely get her disease someday. But since your own marrow wasn't completely normal when it was checked and since you have a high MCV, we check every 6 mos. You're not sick and there's no predicting—absolutely true.

I don't know why I wrote her that day about that. I had told Peter about my situation from the beginning, but, as I said, there was a shadow.

Christmas Day 2016

From Delia to Peter:

Merry Christmas, most darling Peter
Lying in bed reading, eating, mostly longing.
Feeling so lucky and then a jolt, that it's dangerous to say that, inviting a jinx.
But it can't be. Will the besherts (sp.?) protect us?
Hoping I'll never run out of different ways to say I love you.
Your D.

From Peter to Delia:

I am breathless, flattened, limp, longing, at the Best Christmas Greeting/Gift (you) Ever.
There is no jinx, so we don't need the Basherts for that.
Instead they (We) just keep reminding Us that We are All In.
All my love +++++,
Your Peter

We planned a trip after Christmas. We met in Denver and drove south. Six days in a car together. We spent New Year's at a hotel at the Grand Canyon. It was wicked cold and the ground was slippery ice. Peter held me tight as we walked along the trail to the edge and looked down into that vast beautiful world.

part three

Interlude
2017

January and February, we traveled back and forth. I knew stuff about Peter now, like how much he loved to plan and then change plans, that he was obsessed with audiobooks, that he loved to help with everything. If I was craving something four blocks away at ten at night, he was out the door. (This didn't happen often.) We were both tennis fans. He loved any sort of problem to solve.

He pretty much wore the same things when he was not seeing patients: polo shirts with black or blue slacks. Occasionally he wore light blue or blue-striped cotton shirts with collars, the sleeves always messily rolled to his elbows.

He was the only person my age I knew who liked technology. He could fix stuff on my computer. Of course he could—he went to medical school, he had science aptitude, although not a lot, he assured me. He was addicted to his phones. He had two, one work and one personal. Even his son asked him to put them away. He called me "baby-dollsy."

Sometimes I drove him crazy. I would ask if he wanted to do something, and if he hesitated a second, I would answer for him, always negatively: "No? Okay, that's fine."

"I didn't say no," he would say. "I was thinking about it." He objected to my negativity. This happened a lot. I was shocked to realize I was negative, but it was definitely true. I always expected the worst. Was that also from dodging my parents' tirades? I tried to correct over sixty years of that behavior. I warned him not to be optimistic.

Peter was a great listener. He was trained to listen. At the very onset of all our intensity, I warned him that I could drift. Especially when I was writing something. "My mind stays there even when I'm here," I told him. "I can manage not to hear a single thing someone else is saying. I will do this. It will drive you crazy." It did.

It drove Jerry crazy too. I didn't tell Peter that.

*I*n February, Julia's dog Jelly Bean got lost. Jelly was a mostly border collie, dear but somewhat troubled by whatever life she had previous to living in Welsh paradise with Richard and Julia. She bolted out the door of a friend's house, a friend who was keeping her while Julia and Richard were away for the weekend. There was a hunt through the Wye Valley and Monmouth. Jelly's photo was on trees and lampposts. Drones were looking for her. Yes, drones. Also people on horseback, the local huntsman, and many folks in cars. She became, to understate it, everyone's worry. On day three, Julia got word that Jelly had been spotted at Raglan Castle, a medieval castle nine miles away. Julia hurried there and spied her. Julia was not more than seven feet from Jelly, and Jelly bolted as if terrified, tearing away.

Dog trainers got in touch. They explained that fear had made Jelly go feral.

After seven days, when Julia had nearly given up, she heard that Jelly had been spotted near a stream in a small valley. Caroline, Julia's sister, got there first, and, following the advice of one of the dog trainers, she sat with a blanket over her head and a piece of chorizo in her hand held behind her. Jelly crept up and ate the treat. When Julia appeared over the hill and Jelly spotted her, Jelly put her head back and howled like a wolf.

Feral means "returned to an untamed state" or "suggestive of an untamed state." I would think of that much later, after it happened to me.

I am making all sorts of plans for spring and summer. I am hoping we can visit Richard, Julia, and Jelly in May. *Siracusa* is being published in England. I am invited to several UK book festivals. I have a tour for my U.S. paperback in June. There is the speech to the Jungians in Houston in April—it's called "Navigating Life's Absurdities, Obsessions, Hardships." So much to look forward to.

March 13, 2017, the anniversary of Peter's wife's death
From Peter to Delia:

Sweet Delia—
I am so grateful that we have been given our time in life to be together—so poignant at this anniversary time of Virginia's death, and presences all around of Jerry's and Nora's deaths.
All love,
Your P

Delia to Peter:

We are lucky we've been given this time together.
Also it seems more fated than luck.
It's hard to accept the tenderness of it. For me sometimes.
And that is part of the "task"—a weird word to associate with it, but the one I mean because every connection has an obligation even if the obligation is joy—to cherish it.
Very hard to understand how much the deaths of people we love affects us. That is such new territory.
Wish we were on the couch.
All love back, D

$\mathcal{M}$y six-month checkup with Dr. Roboz was on Thursday, March 9. Two days before, I'd noticed two black-and-blue marks on the backs of my calves. I knew from Nora that black-and-blue marks could be a sign of trouble. I photographed them and texted the photo to Dr. Roboz. She told me not to worry.

E-mail to Dr. Roboz, Thursday, March 9, 2017:

> Coming in for blood work. Can I take a Sudafed or Claritin today? Have constant allergies.

From Dr. Roboz to me:

> Yes no problem.

part four

CPX-351

The Center for Blood Disorders at Weill Cornell is on the third floor of the Starr Pavilion. The entrance is on Seventieth Street, between York Avenue and the East River. I travel by subway, thanks to the new Q train, which runs up Second Avenue. I get off at the Sixty-Ninth Street exit and walk two and a half blocks down Seventieth Street, then take one of the crowded small elevators to the third floor.

A large reception area is opposite the elevators. I check in and sit down. I have done this now every six months for eight years. I always notice the variety of folks waiting to see doctors. Every age, every ethnicity, some well dressed, some barely put together. A microcosm of the world. Cancer is an equal opportunity disease. Not that I don't know it, but it's good to realize that I am actually part of a world, even if it's not a world I want to be part of. In fact I assure myself each time I come that I'm not "one of them."

Every time I check in, I'm asked if I have a port or a pick line. I don't exactly know what they are. I don't know that a pick line is actually a PICC line. I say no.

My name is called along with several other patients and we all go for a blood draw.

I should say that I am someone who keeps myself nearly completely medically ignorant. In spite of all the googling I do, I have never googled *myelodysplastic syndrome* or *AML*. If I had to describe leukemia, I would probably say, "Your blood goes crazy, something to do with the white cells." I have e-mails from my sister discussing her disease—intelligently—with words like *blasts* and *cytogenetics*. I know, in some simplistic way, and obviously from context, that those words mean something bad and/or important, but I panic so easily and, in that panic, misunderstand so easily that I try to keep myself in the dark.

Everything else is about to change on this day, but my attitude toward illness will not.

I am called to the small clinic room to see the doctor.

Dr. Roboz's PA (physician's assistant) Evgeny introduces himself and sits at the desk. I have never met one of her PAs in all this time. I say, "I come every six months to have my blood checked. My counts have always been normal."

He is looking at the computer screen, at the results from my blood just taken. "They're not normal," he says hesitantly.

"What?"

He's studying the computer.

Dr. Roboz comes in. He gets up. She sits down and looks.

"It's not normal?" I say.

She tells me something, I don't remember what exactly, to the effect that it could correct. I can come back in a week. As she is sitting there, the rest of the results come in, results that leave no doubt: I have leukemia. I don't remember her telling me. I only remember suddenly knowing it.

She says we have to do a bone marrow biopsy right now.

While they find a room to do it, I call Peter and reach him between patients. He says hello. I say, "I have leukemia."

"We'll get through this," says Peter.

Walking to the subway after the biopsy, I call my dear and brilliant doctor friend Jon and tell him. I call my internist and tell her. She says it could be a mistake and I should come to her office tomorrow and redo the blood work. I reach Peter again between patients. He's flying in tonight on the red-eye.

When I get home, I talk to Peter once more. We agree that when he arrives in the morning, I will have a car pick him up at the airport and we will keep it to go to my internist's later in the morning.

I should say I am aware, writing this now, of the money. Like the cost of sending a car to the airport for Peter and then keeping it for a few hours after. I have made money in my life, not a ton of it, but enough. I know how lucky I am. Every step is a little easier because of it and because I have medical insurance through both the Writers Guild—the screenwriters union—and Medicare.

The news sinks in by me repeating it and repeating it. I don't know who else I call; surely Deena, surely Julia and Jessie. The times between repeating it seem endless and empty.

E-mail to Meredith:

Subject: I'm sorry to put this in an email

The doctors are pretty sure I have leukemia. You know, went for routine blood work and it turned up awful.

Am getting final results Tuesday and am told I should be prepared to go straight into the hospital.

D. xoxo

I knock on Mitch and Stephen's door. They moved into the building after Jerry and me. Mitch, who works in fashion, and Stephen, an interior designer, noticed that I didn't have an office. My desk was in our bedroom. There was a very small room jammed with my files. Stephen said, "Let me turn this into an office for you," and he designed it. Beautiful desk and bookshelves, a wrap-around tackboard for all my research images. Mitch supervised the installation. I begged them to let me pay them for the design and supervision but ended up having to gift them something because Mitch was adamant. "Giving with no expectation of a return is the only way to give," he said. That is, of course, the absolute truth, although I had not thought of it before.

It's been not hard, exactly, but odd, extraordinary, and even blissful to be on the receiving end of Mitch and Stephen's kindnesses.

Thank God these angels live next door to me. Thank God they are home. Mitch hugs me. I spend the evening at their apartment, having dinner with them. We talk about pretty much everything— our families, every catastrophe and happiness in our lives. There is something about my diagnosis that opens our floodgates.

The next morning Peter arrives. He puts his arms around me and I want to disappear into him, just stay there forever.

I get retested and that afternoon learn that the results are the same: unambiguously leukemia. I e-mail Dr. Roboz to tell her I now have black-and-blue marks on my arms. The disease must be progressing. She tells me she will call on Saturday when she sees the results of my bone marrow biopsy.

I am sitting on the couch in my bedroom when she calls, a fact that has no particular significance except I think you always remember where you are when you get bad news. She confirms it: I have AML. This illness presents differently in different people, she tells me, and mine is not like Nora's. "You are not your sister" is a refrain she and Jon drum into me again and again, willing me to believe that I can have a different outcome. Dr. Roboz and Jon speak often throughout my illness (with my consent, of course). Dr. Roboz says there is a new drug, in the final stages of testing, that she thinks is absolutely suited to me: CPX-351.

The magic potion. CPX-351. I don't google it. But I have hope.

I will check into the hospital on Tuesday.

I have lists in my computer of all the appointments I have to cancel. Simple things like dinners. The Jungian conference. They need a reason. Julia has a problem with her eye. I borrow her disease. Neither of my screenplays require rewrites now, so I can put a hold on those. (Although one note I write says, *Ask Jessie for help on act 2.* Somewhere I must believe life will go on.) I can't see Heather or baby Rowan. For how long, I don't know. I can't expose myself to babies or young children. My immune system is flattened. A cold or flu could kill me.

Meredith, my friend in San Francisco, wise about all things medical, e-mails me a list of things to pack for my weeks-long hospital stay. Linda, my housekeeper, who worked for Nora forever and still works for Nora's husband, Nick, and is like family, agrees to care for Honey as well as me. She will come to the hospital often. I know she will be comforting. I decide Peter and I need a sofa bed in case anyone stays in the apartment to visit or whatever. Mitch makes the purchase and is happy to supervise its arrival. He also gifts me an entire hospital wardrobe—soft T-shirts, sweats, a shawl, sweaters, and socks.

Jon and his wife, Kate, ask Peter and me to dinner Saturday night. They are the warmest couple, and Jon is the busiest man. In addition to having a family and his private medical practice, he broadcasts regularly on CBS, flies all over the place for stories, and runs our Empathy Project. Still, he shows up when it matters, not just for me but for all his friends. He and Kate know this prehospitalization weekend will be full of anxiety. I am safe at their home, comforted.

All these are godsends that come to me from friends.

Sudden catastrophe changes everything. Peter is going to take a leave of absence from his practice to be with me.

I have told the ten or so people who know not to tell anyone else, and I believe they are trustworthy. I am not suited to secrets, I know that, but if this news is batted around publicly, people may give up on me, reduce me to *Her sister died. She's dying too.* Dr. Roboz and Jon want me to believe I will be okay. "You are not your sister." This is the mantra. The nature of my AML is different from Nora's, they tell me again and again. My marrow is different. I can have a different outcome. They believe that I need to believe that and understand that. They repeat it again and again.

So, ironically, like Nora but unlike me, I keep my illness secret.

I could probably have an entire analysis based on the idea that I will survive if I believe I am not my sister. As a child, I simply tried to do everything she did, although she was going around the track so fast, I couldn't keep up. Writing taught me who I was, because your writing is your fingerprint. When I began to do it, I heard my own voice, my own observations, my own stories, my own gifts. Although we were always close and occasional collaborators, I valued our differences. But I loved her. And now believing that I'm not like her seems almost a betrayal. Yet it could save me.

On Sunday morning, Peter is at the kitchen table and I am making us French toast. Peter says, "We should get married."

Then, I suspect because he's hearing his own words, he stands up and says, "Will you marry me?"

"Yes," I say.

Later I asked him about it: Why the proposal then? He said we both knew we would one day get married, and sitting there at the breakfast table, knowing what was coming at us, he suddenly realized, yes, we should do it now.

It isn't romantic. I mean, I'm holding a spatula in my hand, feeling terror about my diagnosis, about the next weeks, my future, our future, but "We should get married" feels absolutely right.

Monday, the day before my hospitalization, we take a taxi to that big building on Worth Street, the Office of the City Clerk, and get a marriage license. And then we stop in to see Ron at my local antique-jewelry shop and buy a ring, a woven platinum band.

Tuesday I check in. Linda goes with me. Peter has flown back to California to put his life and practice in order. He comes back Friday and never leaves again.

I am officially a cancer patient now, a leukemia patient. My life is not mine anymore. Hospitals are not prisons, obviously, but you live by their rules. Before I can have this chemotherapy, I have my heart and lungs scanned. I learn about PICC lines because I get one. PICC: a peripherally inserted central catheter. It's a skinny tube inserted into a vein in my left upper arm. The end goes into a central vein near my heart so that the nurse doesn't need to stick a needle in me every time she or he takes blood or gives me a chemo infusion. The nurses do take my blood every day.

When the first tech tries to insert the PICC line, I writhe and scream. They bring in another tech, who inserts it swiftly and painlessly. One of the many things I learn in hospitals is that there is often someone who can do a procedure better. If it doesn't go well at first, you can ask for someone else to try it. I like to become expert in things. I love to think, *Oh, I can tell this to a friend.* This part of me is still operating. There are so many levels operating— the same old Delia, trying to learn and get better at anything new; the frightened Delia who thinks her life might be over; the Delia who is madly in love.

Peter meets Dr. Roboz. Afterward, he tells me, "We are on the Roboz train. We go wherever she tells us." And somewhere in here, I tell Dr. Roboz that she doesn't need to inform me of everything. The way the disease may or may not progress—the science and odds of all this are not something I want in my brain. She hears me.

But she can tell Peter things, because I have given her permission, and, besides, he has my medical power of attorney. I know, even though he says we follow her lead, that Peter will track my blood counts and everything else. He's a doctor. I'm marrying a doctor.

I am aware that I am lucky. It's a bit pathetic to be dealt one of the worst cards in the deck and still try to find some way to believe that you are lucky. But that part of me is operating too. I know it is good to have this illness diagnosed early, to have my oncologist in place. I can imagine how deranged I would be if I were hunting for one now, exploring treatments.

I can spend the first week on the expensive floor, says Dr. Roboz. This is the fourteenth floor of the Greenberg Pavilion, where you pay a lot extra for a private room, can order good food, and the views are pretty. I know this floor well. I have had friends convalesce here. My sister died here. Then I will move to the tenth floor, Ten North, where the serious oncology takes place, and the nurses are Dr. Roboz's nurses. I know this floor too. Dr. Roboz promises not to put me in Nora's rooms.

Peter and I tell Dr. Roboz we want to get married on Saturday.

As a result, two chaplains pay a visit. Dr. Cheryl Fox, the one who will be at the hospital that day, agrees to read the vows and sign the license. My friend Jessie will perform the ceremony.

Peter tells his kids we are getting married. They are sweet about it. Sympathetic.

I invite a very few close friends, mostly by e-mail, a few by phone—only those who know I'm sick—to come to our wedding in the private dining room on the fourteenth floor of the hospital this Saturday at two.

It's a sunny day. Light streams in the dining-room window. Jessie, funny and compassionate, is very good at weddings. She tells our story, which she knows not only from the e-mails we sent her but also from my calling her every single second in the beginning, worrying my head off, asking for advice.

In the photos Jon takes, all the guests—in a semicircle around Peter and me—are smiling and some are wiping away tears. I am pale and have a scrunched-up tissue clutched in one hand and a bunch of daffodils in the other. My arm is through Peter's, holding him tight, and his free hand is on mine. I'm wearing a white silk blouse and slacks and my gorgeous red suede shoes with gold heels. On my wrist I wear my hospital band and an enamel bracelet, a present from my neighbors Mitch and Stephen.

In the service Jessie includes Peter's favorite quote from Jung: "The meeting of two personalities is like the contact of two chemical substances. If there is any reaction, both are transformed."

Jessie hands out candles, long white tapers. Peter lights his, I light mine from his, Jessie lights hers from mine, and so forth—the flame is passed around the room. Jessie asks our guests: "Do you vow to hold and guide Delia and Peter to the better angels of their natures?" Everyone together says, "I do."

Then Cheryl Fox, the chaplain, takes over. We read our vows, which Peter has written. Peter's voice is strong.

"I, Peter, take you, Delia, to have and to hold, to love and to cherish, and to heck with the rest of that traditional vow, which we replace with our certainty of navigating the miraculous life stream of the Bashert that has brought us together—a miracle in itself that shall only beget the next miracle and the next. I love you very much, Delia mine."

My vow is the same, reversing the names, of course. My voice is weak and teary. I cry through mine.

Peter kisses the ring before he slips it on my finger.

We have my favorite layer cakes from Amy's Bread—chocolate with white frosting and yellow with pink frosting. Jessie picked them up—they weigh quite a lot—and in the rush to get here and also to hunt for a Staples to have our vows xeroxed, she tripped and fell. She managed somehow to hold on to the beautiful cakes but ripped a huge hole in her tights, which fortunately no one notices. The hospital chef provides a delicious lemon meringue pie. I love everyone in the room. I have had the first of three treatments. CPX-351 is purple. It looks like Kool-Aid. The infusion takes ninety minutes.

Looking now at the photos, I am reminded how Peter and our friends showered me with love. I believe it was powerful. Probably every person at the wedding knew my chances were slim. But none of them brought that feeling with them. It was a room full of hope.

$\mathcal{T}$he way CPX works: I get three infusions, with a day between each. The hope is that this chemotherapy will clean out my marrow, kill off the cells, especially all the cancerous white cells, and only healthy white cells will grow in their place. I get blood drawn every morning, and depending on the results, I may get a transfusion, red cells or platelets, because they go very low too. My blood is now an ever-changing entity.

It's really hard and rare to transfuse white cells, which protect from infection. If I get a fever, Dr. Roboz will have to douse me with antibiotics and hope for the best. My few visitors can't come if they or anyone they live with has a sniffle. They have to Purell their hands in the hallway. They sit well across the room. It is strange to be fragile—it's a disconnect to think of myself that way, as someone from whom people have to keep their distance. It's actually freakish. But then, having a possibly fatal cancer has made me immediately "other."

For the first ten days or so after the infusions begin, I feel fine. I'm not totally fine, of course, because I have leukemia. Nurses come at regular intervals to check my blood pressure and oxygen and take my temperature. Also, CPX has side effects. One day, I stand up and my legs crumple; I clutch the bed, breaking my fall. Many medical people come to evaluate me. Jessie is there that afternoon, as well as Peter. I tell her she can leave and she says calmly, "I think I'll stay awhile longer," and I realize, *Oh, she's worried about me.*

Of course she is. I knew it before, but there is something about this moment that makes it more real, if there actually is such a thing as "more real." *Jessie is worried. My friends are worried.* Peter begins sending e-mail updates to my close friends and family. I learn later that Alice starts e-mailing Julia and Deena. She gets their e-mail addresses off Peter's updates. They all share their concerns and my medical news. They have heard about one another from me over the years—Deena in Pasadena, Alice in Berkeley, Julia in Wales. Now they are friends.

What I don't remember during this time is discussing death with Peter, but it's a presence. One night I have the strongest feeling that Jerry and Nora are there with me, and I worry they have come to take me away. I have nightmares—about being lost in dangerous places, cliffs and canyons. In the only one I remember clearly, there is a huge rock mountain blocking my path, and then it cracks slightly, letting in a sliver of light. I tell Peter about it. (Jungians are great believers in dreams.) Although I am frightened in the dream, Peter says it's a dream of hope—that crack is my way through. There will be a way out.

My chances of survival depend on this drug. *Dr. Roboz is positive. She believes it can work. I am a good candidate. Maybe she's right. Peter is positive, always positive. You are not your sister.* It's all banging around in my head every day. All the time, every day.

One morning, leaving the bathroom, I suddenly pass out. My head hits the floor. I am out for only a second. I open my eyes to see Peter over me, and he says with the regret that is instantly on both our minds, "I guess we have to tell them."

There could be bleeding in my brain, says Dr. Roboz. I am wheeled down for an MRI. Thank God, I'm fine.

We walk the hallways, my arm in Peter's, and radiate so much affection that nurses and orderlies randomly ask us how long we've been married, thinking we will say, *Fifty years.* At our age, we are everyone's fantasy of long enduring romantic love. We tell them three days, a week, two weeks.

This time would be boring—actually, it is boring. A blur of people taking my vital signs, meals arriving I don't want to eat—but at the same time it's not boring because I'm scared. It's both repetitive— the routine, that is—and unpredictable. I don't remember reading books. That level of concentration is beyond me. We watch cheery things on TV, like *Schitt's Creek.* The hospital lets Peter use a small business room so he can continue to see his patients by phone or Zoom. I think this helps him remember who he is. Without being able to practice, he could lose himself, because, aside from his seeing patients and checking in by phone with his kids, his vigilance is constant. He sleeps on a daybed here every night.

I don't know how he can do it, really. I remember when Jerry was in the hospital. Around seven or eight every night, after a day there, I would feel that I absolutely had to get out. I had to get home. Peter occasionally goes to our apartment, but he says his home is where I am. Perhaps some of this stamina is his medical training, the hours he spent years ago on overnight call. Mostly, I think, it's love. The freshness of our love.

Every night he makes up the daybed in the room. Before I fall asleep, I always see Peter across the way, reading, waiting for me to fall asleep before he does. Sometimes, illegally, he slips into my bed, hoping the nurses won't catch us. Which they don't. I love having his arms around me, feeling his body next to mine. I love the silliness of the sneak. Peter buoys me. And he's my protective shield.

When Peter does need a break or is working, Linda is here. Linda is one of the smartest, most loving people I know. Her life has been extraordinary. At fourteen years of age, she survived a brutal earthquake in Managua, Nicaragua, that killed her cousins, who were sleeping in the room with her. The house collapsed and she crawled out of the wreckage, pulling her younger boy cousin with her, saving both their lives. At fifteen, she crossed the Mexico-U.S. border and joined her mother in New York City. She learned to speak English fluently, raised her three children, and became an American citizen while she worked for Nora and then for me as well. She took a break to get a nursing degree, worked awhile at that, and came back to us. She decided she was happier working for us. We certainly were.

During this illness, she is my mother. She brings warmth and love and she makes sure I do things like brush my teeth. No one has had to remind me of that since I was maybe six years old, but it's amazing how easy it is in the hospital to lose my daily routine and sink into a kind of lazy despair.

I discover that I can disappear from "normal" life for a month (actually, it's five weeks) and no one notices. I don't remember e-mailing anyone outside my bubble other than, occasionally, businesspeople to answer questions. I write Marian, the publicist at Blue Rider Press who is booking my paperback tour for *Siracusa* in June, that I "may have to have a medical procedure," and it would be wise to book refundable fares. What I really mean is I may be dead. There is an anxious e-mail from my editor saying how important my tour is. I can't tell anyone there how sick I am. It's a small publishing imprint, about ten people; everyone who works there is close and friendly. *Siracusa* had good hardcover sales and a movie option. My paperback tour matters to them. But if I secretly tell the editor in chief, how can he not tell my editor? One will confide in another who will confide in another. I don't want to be doomed before I have a chance to live. I feel the most guilty about keeping my illness from them, but it seems like the only way to go.

I have to protect my hope.

There is a whole thing about staying clean. I'm supposed to wash all over my body with chlorhexidine, a powerful antiseptic. I turn out to be allergic to it, and my skin shreds. Pretty much all my skin. Not like a snake, not in whole big pieces, just constant shredding all over.

I wear a wristband declaring this allergy.

And, of course, I'm not allowed flowers.

It's strange, isn't it? Something that can cure me makes flowers dangerous. What can a flower possibly do to me? A flower. Somehow that says it all about how chemo is a poison cure.

We are told that if the CPX is working, after ten days, all my blood counts will topple. Dr. Roboz orders a bone marrow biopsy to see what's happening.

In the meantime, with my marrow fragile, I am more vulnerable to infection and bleeding. I have been moved to the oncology floor in anticipation of this. The oncology floor was where Nora got all her bad news. As I am being pushed there in a wheelchair, I am thinking, *Please don't put me in her room, please. How can I believe I am not my sister if I am in her room?* Did Dr. Roboz remember my request? I'm too scared to ask. They wheel me into a nice corner room. A wave of relief. I am extremely grateful.

The fourteenth floor has lovely river and city views. It's odd how things true about life when you are healthy are even truer when you are not. Light makes me feel better; it makes me happier—a sunny day, a sunset, a view of the Fifty-Ninth Street Bridge. Ten North, on the other hand, feels gray, a serious place where I am more seriously ill. One night, very late, my heart starts palpitating. Peter takes my pulse. It's racing. The night physician's assistant is summoned. They can't find the doctor. Peter gets angry. I have never seen him angry. He's fierce. "I want the doctor for my wife." I watch from the bed. Peter refuses to back down to the PA and nurses. It is odd to realize it is for me—that I am in danger. There is some way—this is probably common—that I protect myself from understanding how sick I am. It's as if his anger might be for someone else. This is similar to my sudden awareness that Jessie was worried. But more powerful, because it is Peter.

They locate the doctor. Peter talks to him on the phone. The doctor puts me on a new medication, and the nurses hook me up to a heart monitor. At some central location, far from the hospital, my heartbeat is now being tracked twenty-four hours a day along with the fragile hearts of many other patients.

I am soon told that I have atrial fibrillation—an irregular heartbeat—and prescribed a pill to take daily. A-fib is a complication of treatment. It can cause blood clots or strokes. But not, hopefully, if I take a pill.

E-mail from Peter to Julia and Deena:

> We were just told that Delia's first round of chemo brought the best possible result, so we are way out ahead on beating this! Dr. Roboz could not be more pleased, and thus are we!

The marrow has been "emptied out" of all cells, and odds are excellent that only healthy cells will grow back, with the next indicators in about 10 days.

We know that the love and life energy we are all sharing (confluencing?) is helping bring this about!

Thanks for taking such good care of my wife, and one another, as we're just getting started.

Love, Peter

My blood counts begin to rise again, as they are supposed to after about twelve days. They keep climbing. The question now is, will the new white cells be healthy?

I am released from the hospital after a five-week stay without knowing the answer to this question. It's spring. The few trees along Seventieth Street are blossoming. It's remarkable to feel a breeze.

I am uncertain outside. Street confidence—after weeks in the hospital on chemotherapy—is blown. I don't have it. The city is always full of distractions, but especially in the spring when everybody rediscovers the outdoors. I love April in New York, but now I feel fragile, looking every which way before I cross a street. I walk two blocks to meet Jessie for dinner and am anxious the entire time. Although Jessie, who has a calm otherworldly certainty about things, tells me that when she saw me walking toward her, she thought, *She's going to be all right.*

When Peter and I are out together, he always holds my arm. One morning on our way into Washington Square Park, where the cherry and magnolia trees are bursting with bright pink blossoms, I can't figure out why Peter is tense. I mean, it's gorgeous here, but he is glancing every which way. "What are you looking for?" I ask.

"I'm looking for any people or dogs who could crash into you. I'm trying to keep you safe," he says.

Is he replaying his trauma from childhood? He couldn't save his mother. He was outside, he was nearby, but he wasn't looking. And, my God, he was seven. He was playing with friends. Now he's twisting in every direction at once. He's not letting anything happen to me. He tells me, "I'm your guardian beagle."

I don't really want to go anywhere. In fact, I could spend the rest of my life inside, but Peter suggests the opera. My first opera. My blood counts are good. We are told it is safe. Linda tells me I should do this. "This would be good for you," she says. So I go to the Met for the first time.

The Metropolitan Opera. A truly elegant New York thing that I know only from the movies. Mostly from Cher in *Moonstruck,* looking spectacularly glamorous after a montage involving shopping, makeup, and hair. She waits at the Lincoln Center fountain for Nicolas Cage to arrive and introduce her to love and life with her first night at the opera. I don't actually remember which opera is in that movie, but I remember Cher.

I dress up, I even wear a skirt, and the interior of the theater is beautiful, all deep red and gold. Because I am not yet at full strength—and operas can be long—we leave after the first act. It is like visiting another country, full of New Yorkers more cultured than me. Peter loves the opera. Dr. Roboz loves it. Ruth Bader Ginsburg loved it. I've read that about her. I want to say that I love it too—I am happy to go again, anything to make Peter happy—but I can say only that I love people who love the opera.

Peter to Alice, Deena, and Julia, Saturday, April 15:

I know that Delia has been in touch with each of you with news that we are home since Monday, with Delia feeling increasingly like herself despite the ordeal of it all, with white counts returning to normal. Delia is stronger by the day, and we are taking several daily walks in the beautiful neighborhood. She is gradually recovering her appetite and taste buds, providing wonderful spontaneous whims of what she would like to eat, although her own home-made grilled cheese sandwiches remain both the highlight and the benchmark. The all-important next bone marrow biopsy should tell us if this is a true remission and will be drawn this Monday morning, and we should know the results a few days later.

Oh, and we went to the Met Opera two nights ago to hear the new production premiere of *Der Rosenkavalier*, with Renée Fleming (first act only, please, a good 1 hour and 13 minutes, but full of great beauty). We are watching some baseball, and missing *Schitt's Creek* now that we've finished it. I must admit in introducing each other to our different interests that Stanley Cup hockey playoffs are a tougher sell than opera!

Thanks for all the love and the hope and the healing energies!

Love, Peter (and for Delia)

$\mathcal{T}$he all-important next bone marrow biopsy," as Peter called it—Natalie does this one. She is Dr. Roboz's other PA. There are two—Evgeny Mikler, enthusiastic and warm, and Natalie Tafel, deliberate and charming. On the staff, there is also Irene Gerahty, who schedules everything, as well as Michelle Patrice and Virginia Hernandez, always upbeat and friendly, who run the clinic. I always think that one way you can judge doctors is by the people who work under them. Roboz's team is positive and kind, and they never act like Dr. Roboz should be protected from her patients. Or that I should be in awe of her. Although I am.

Natalie is very good at this awful thing, bone marrow biopsies. From now on, I will request her.

I close my eyes and lie on my stomach with my hands above my head so Peter can hold them to comfort me. Natalie taps my hip looking for a good place, whatever that is, then gives me a warning and a quick shot of a local anesthetic. I open my eyes to see if Peter is watching, thinking he will be a curious, dispassionate doctor, because one of the most shocking things I know about Peter is this: he had two colonoscopies without anesthetic (because he wanted to watch and he wanted to drive himself home).

His eyes are squeezed shut.

In spite of the numbing, when Natalie sticks a larger needle into my bone to extract the marrow, it's painful. Some bone marrow biopsies hurt much more than others, and it's hard to know why. But everyone dreads them. Natalie narrates every move she makes and cheers when she extracts the tissue and it's over.

Several days later, Peter and I wait nervously in the clinic room to hear results.

Dr. Roboz bursts in. "Your marrow is gorgeous."

part five

Dark Clouds
Part

*R*emission.

Impossible to underestimate the power of that word.

Peter and I are instantly imagining and planning a future.

We buy a Ping-Pong table. This may not seem like the most obvious next move, but we wander into a furniture store—the dangers of loving to walk in Manhattan—and stumble across a handsome Ping-Pong table, black with very cool slanted legs. It's slightly smaller than a regular one. There are two racquets and a ball, and we have so much fun playing in the store, we buy it. In order to fit it into the apartment, we squeeze the dining-room table into the living room and stick the Ping-Pong table in the dining room. It's pretty ridiculous but it instantly makes my apartment ours.

The first thing Peter does when we wake up in the morning is wrap his arms around me. I snuggle into his shoulder. It's the moment in the day when I am happiest. When death is farthest away.

I think about it all the time. Sometimes very consciously, and sometimes it's just fluttering in the back of things. For me, that is the most stunning thing about remission—the glorious sense that I have been given back life coupled with the terrible fear that death is behind the next lamppost. This gift could be snuffed out at any moment.

Life and death in close focus, side by side.

The average remission for CPX is fourteen months. Who tells me that? I have no idea. It must be Dr. Roboz. I seem to block out the moments when crucial and agitating information is given to me. I retain the information but not the delivery of it. I also mishear information, as you will see. In any event, fourteen months is the average. Maybe I will get more, much more. Many people with cancer have lasted way longer than expected, I tell myself, although I can't really come up with anyone except a friend of a friend.

Peter and Meredith both assure me there are many new drugs for AML. When this one stops working, Dr. Roboz, who is cutting-edge in her knowledge of and access to treatments, will find another. I'm living on what many cancer patients live on: the promise of science. CPX was in final testing. Some other drug will be too.

My blood is now under constant care. With AML, remission does not mean "Go live your life and have a checkup every few months." My illness is my life.

I have to go to Weill Cornell for a blood draw once or twice a week, depending on the counts. I can't take subways because I cannot risk getting sick. I love subways—the efficiency, the speed, the absolute New York of them—but now I'm told to consider them danger zones. I can't risk getting the flu. The flu will become pneumonia, and with my injured immune system, that will be the end of me. I'm not sure why my odds of survival are better in a rackety New York City taxi on the FDR Drive, but I follow instructions.

This is my routine at the hospital. I get off the elevator, usually with Peter, and check in at the computer, then at the desk. "Do you have a port or PICC line?" "A PICC line," I answer.

I am now like almost all the patients—in treatment. I don't mind that I'm "one of them," that others are surviving and struggling, that we're all in it together. Yet, of course, each of us is absolutely and completely alone. A possibly fatal disease is an isolation cell.

They do a blood draw. Some days my counts are low and I need a transfusion, red blood cells or platelets, which means I have to wait for the blood to arrive. Sometimes I get into arguments with the staff because it doesn't come for hours. When it does, I sit, usually with Peter, in a small space with a little curtain, outfitted with a comfortable chair and a TV. There are rows of these cubicles all filled with people getting something intravenously. The nurses appear and there is a big double check—they recite the order to each other confirming that I am me and I'm getting the blood I'm supposed to.

First they give me Zofran, whatever that is, so I don't get nauseous. Very nice volunteers come around. One day I get a free blanket from Subaru. Two young women offering cancer patients information on makeup catch me watching *Law & Order: SVU*. "Is this what you're watching?" one says with dismay. I deny it. I act as if the TV has landed on that channel by accident.

I don't know if it's the chemotherapy or the possibly fatal diagnosis or the uncertainty inherent in remission or all of those things, but my relationship to the world has changed. It's as if I've been knocked on the head. I look the same, I think, although there is uncertainty in my reflection that wasn't there before. Would anyone else notice that? I'm not sure. I am physically, mentally, and emotionally wobbly.

As soon as it's safe, I go to Eugene for a blow-dry. CPX, amazingly, does not make a person's hair fall out.

I've been going to Eugene for twelve years. I've followed him from one salon to another. I think he is touched by the spirits. I always leave calmer, and not simply because I have good hair— although let's not underestimate the importance of that. He is positive—relaxed positive. Innately kind and decent. I have never seen him in a bad mood. He grew up in Washington, DC, and, as many talented people do, he found his way to New York City, which he loves as much as I do. I am his oldest client. I don't mean in age, although that may be possible. I mean I've been seeing him longer than anyone else.

I met him when, needing a blow-dry, I walked into a random salon in my neighborhood, looked around, and there he was: the most cool, tall young Black man with Rastafarian braids.

One day he decided he needed to see the world, and—while still doing hair, thank God—he spent the next couple of years traveling in short spurts, constantly and curiously. A few days here, a week there; Greece, Italy, Paris, the UK, Israel, Tokyo, Argentina, to name a few. Then he stopped. Now he's baking cakes on the side, decorated and delicious fantasy creations. They are works of art. His clients are begging to order them, but he's selective. For one thing, he works full-time. I told him before I went into the hospital that I had leukemia. We were walking down the salon stairs to check out, and he nodded and squeezed my shoulder. I knew he was upset. I knew he wouldn't want to upset me.

I won't discuss my horrible curls and how Eugene makes them behave and no one else ever has, but my attachment to him is big. I confide to Eugene that Peter and I are married. We discuss whether Peter and I will have a party when I decide to tell people news of that and of my illness. A wedding reception. "Will you bake the cake?"

"Yes," he says. "How should I decorate it?"

"I'm figuring that out. Roses, for sure; memories—maybe Peter's Subaru that we traveled around in, maybe the Grand Canyon." I am thinking big here.

All these different friendships. Mine with Eugene is both business and personal. These bonds matter. They are little homes. Places of safety. I am taking stock now. Friendship. God, I love my friends.

One day, on my way to Eugene, I get out of the cab at Twenty-Third Street, cross Eighth Avenue to the west side of the street, and my legs buckle. They give out. Thank God, there is a lamppost. I grab it. I wait a minute, holding on, assessing. My legs seem okay. I let go and walk to the salon.

I move around gingerly inside, wondering if it's going to happen again, holding tight to the railing when I go to the second floor.

This legs-giving-out thing starts to happen frequently, sometimes at home when I stand up, but mostly when I get out of a cab. Since I'm not allowed on the subway, there are lots of those episodes. I give it a name: taxi legs. Dr. Roboz can't explain it. She counsels me to "rise up slowly" and "give yourself a second before you take off. Try to take note of your heart rate (does it feel like it's racing?)." It doesn't. And "make sure you are keeping well-hydrated." Drinking water becomes an urgent thing—I have to do it all day, every day.

I get black streaks across my nails. Dr. Roboz explains that this is similar to the way trees get rings around them, evidence of trauma. I also get chills and often wear a jacket or coat when I'm inside.

Peter starts to accompany me to the salon whenever possible, whenever he doesn't have patients. He's good-humored about it, waiting for me on the couch, listening to an audiobook. Sometimes he walks over to Sullivan Street Bakery on Ninth Avenue and buys us their delicious cold pizza. We shop together at our local market. We look, I suppose, like every retired couple I saw when I was lively, healthy, and about thirty. *The two of them don't have anything to do,* I would think, with a young person's arrogance, *except discuss whether to buy frozen spinach.* But maybe I was wrong. Maybe she had a fatal disease and he, worried, didn't want her to shop alone. Maybe they had just fallen in love and couldn't bear to be apart. Maybe they simply adored the supermarket, with all its products and possibilities. Maybe they were just friends. Old age and its many varieties were beyond me then.

I have been wanting to visit the apartment building on Central Park West where Peter lived until he was twelve. Most specifically, I want to reimagine the transforming event of his life. He has been through so much trauma with me in such a short time. Going there is a way to honor his scars.

We take a taxi up to Central Park West and 102nd Street. The building, facing the park, is unchanged, Peter says—a bulky, almost funky, 1902 beaux arts building with a wavy facade and curved corners. An arched entry in the center links two large ten-story structures.

It's quiet. A sunny, cold day. The street looks absolutely the same as it did sixty-six years ago. Trees probably larger, cars parked bumper to bumper along the park side, newer cars—those are the only differences. Peter shows me where he was playing after school with his friends while his mother was talking with the other moms, where his mom and his sister crossed the street, stepping out between two parked cars. Where he heard an otherworldly, loud screech. Where he saw them lying bloody on the street in front of the car that hit them.

Peter tells me more about that afternoon. He was carried home by Bella, his mother's best friend, who also lived in the building. She had him call his dad. I try to imagine at seven years old calling your father to tell him this news. His father took a long time to get there. "What took you so long?" Peter sobbed.

"I took the subway, it's faster," said his dad.

As if that were the question—subway versus taxi. *I've been all alone* was what Peter was saying but in his distress couldn't articulate. *I'm scared.*

For Peter, looking back, it was the first time he understood the coolness of his father's heart.

There is no evidence out here on the sidewalk or street of this tragedy sixty-six years ago. No memorial, no marker. Peter walked outside every day past this spot until they moved to Cincinnati five years later. Until then, he still played here every day either with his friends or by himself, endlessly throwing his pink Spaldeen against the building wall and narrating made-up Dodgers games.

I ask him what it was like to continue living and playing here where this tragedy happened.

He thinks about it awhile. "I just did it," he says. "That's what you do with trauma. You tamp it down. It was the street where I lived."

$\mathcal{P}$eter takes a short trip to California.

He sees his kids, their mates, his granddaughter, his patients, and finds us a new place to live that suits me more: a tiny one-bedroom in a five-story elevator apartment building on the main street of San Rafael. Then he takes another trip back to actually make the move and see his patients in person again.

San Rafael is a sweet, small city about a half hour north of San Francisco over the Golden Gate Bridge. A mix of races and classes. I fall in love with it in a tour Peter gives me on FaceTime. I can walk within seconds to everything—restaurants; a great sandwich shop; cappuccinos; many blow-dry choices; pizza; a refurbished art deco movie theater; a Copperfield's bookstore that sells not only books but chocolate chip cookies; a pet-supply store (should Honey ever travel with us); a sporting-goods store; an electronics store; even a place that sells old coins. Right out the door—there it all is. I'm taking Peter away from his redwoods of Mill Valley, but it's our new life together and he is happy. We take a year's lease, a stake in the future.

Our new apartment is, most excellently, five minutes from Naftali, Alyson, and little Idra.

I prefer an apartment to an isolated condo, cityscapes to residential neighborhoods. I like other people living stacked up around me. Peter FaceTimes me from our little home on the top floor and shows me its sunny view of green Marin County hills and the San Rafael Mission.

I like to drive. I grew up in the flats of Beverly Hills. Turn me loose anywhere in Los Angeles, and I'm fine, but I know nothing of the streets and highways around San Francisco and Marin County. I'm not planning to master that tangle. A walking city gives me more options.

This is a concession to age, the first thing I won't do because I'm old. Well, there are a million things I won't do, that I would never do, like parachute jumping and whitewater rafting. Truthfully, I am and have always been a scaredy-cat. Being alone in a house at night makes me nervous. This has been true from childhood. But not driving here—this is the first thing I'm not doing because I'm old. Or maybe it's not that. Perhaps I'm frightened, jarred by the illness. Jarred by the cure. Maybe the illness threw me into old age. Maybe that's why I can no longer muster the nerve to drive. Although, when I despair about this to Meredith, my San Francisco friend who is especially smart about all things medical, she kindly points out that there are all different ways to be brave. My curiosity is blunted now. My adventurousness. Remission is a gorgeous but temporary refuge. The larger fear—the cancer returning—has so rattled me, I want to keep everything simple, all risks to a minimum.

During Peter's visits west, he tells his patients he has married and is moving to New York. He will be happy to do sessions on the phone or on Zoom (a secure video feed that almost nobody knew about then). He will be back and forth for a while, but in a couple of months he will let his offices in San Francisco and Mill Valley go. If patients want to leave him but continue with therapy, he promises to find them psychotherapists they like and who will take their insurance. My cancer has completely changed both our lives.

Peter doesn't mind this. He doesn't agonize over it. He was planning to retire in two years, and he is a guy who has changed his life and his cities before. He sends his twenty volumes of Carl Jung's *Collected Works* east. We clear a bookshelf for them above the couch in what is now Peter's office. On the shelf he also puts a lovely framed photo of his granddaughter. We start to eat dinner there, with our food on a piano bench in front of the couch. Also, Peter tapes up a twelve-month calendar featuring photos of the Southwest, views of Arches National Park, Bryce Canyon, and the like. He needs those visuals. He loves them. He sticks the calendar on the office closet door with bright blue electrician's tape.

We don't have the need or energy to re-create or reimagine our lives more. These changes are enough for us. We are deeply together, how is less important. Death is knocking at the door.

Peter is great at running things. The apartment, the repairs. He books trips, tickets, dinner reservations, always consulting me about what I would like to do, where I would like to go. You might be thinking this is too good to be true, but it is actually unnerving. With Jerry, I organized our life, although in an old-school fashion. We both paid bills by check and made dinner reservations by phone. I made sure the air-conditioning was serviced and tracked other house stuff like that. What money we had, to the extent it needed managing, I managed it. But while my remission may be a relief, it is not peaceful. My brain is too jumbled with anxiety to do things that need focus and concentration, like pay bills and track our accounts. And I am way behind the times. I don't even understand Venmo and Zelle. I ask Peter to take over, and he moves everything online with great efficiency.

This is a huge change in my relationship to the world. An overwhelming relief. And beyond pleasant. Although what worries me is, if something happens to Peter, I will be riding in a car without a driver.

I have two unsettling dinners when Peter is away. First with Louisa.

Louisa is a writer and magazine editor who lives on Prince Street just south of Greenwich Village in SoHo. She was also born on Prince Street when it was strictly an Italian neighborhood. She is completely rooted in her Italian past. Her husband died about thirteen years ago, and she has been advising me on life-after. The ends of her pale blond hair are tinted pink or lavender. She leaves fantastic tips, always in cash, and drinks things like vodka straight. She names the brand. I'm good for maybe a half a glass of wine. Tonight I pretend to drink. I order it and look at it. My internist told me that alcohol is bad for my bone marrow. Dr. Roboz doesn't say that, but my internist has spooked me.

I met Louisa through Julia. They met at the Sharjah International Book Fair, an event in the United Arab Emirates. Julia gave a talk, translated into Arabic, to white-robed men who, Julia said, "looked mystified." Only Julia or Louisa would go someplace like this. They are both literary, game, and great travelers. Julia said, "Oh my God, my best friend lives right near you," so I met Louisa.

Louisa doesn't know I've been sick. She doesn't know I'm

remarkably different, emotionally and actually, from the last time
we had dinner. She doesn't know I'm married.

I pretend to be who I was. We talk about being single after losing
our husbands. We talk about dating at this age. We talk about Peter
as if I'm dating him. She says she hopes I bought great lingerie.
We discuss her Syrian writer boyfriend in Berlin with whom she's
off and on again. When we leave, Louisa tucks her arm in mine as
we walk along Ninth Street, and I am panicking that she's going to
feel my PICC line. The port to it pokes out on my left inner arm.
She is going to say, *What is this?* Or, worse, she's going to know
what it is.

I feel, after this dinner, a sense of dishonesty—that I am not a
friend. I am pretending to be a friend.

I also have dinner with Lisa and Marie. Lisa knows I've been sick,
but Marie doesn't. Marie is a brilliant investigative journalist up on
every single thing happening—politics, society, writers, medicine,
crime, money, the famous, the near famous, name it. Some of the
time I'm not sure whom she is talking about or referring to—
I am not inclined to be as engaged in the world as she is—but I
always leave dinner wiser. And she is generous, beyond generous,
and so happy for her friends when good things happen to them.
I have known her for forty years, since I first came to New York
to become a writer. Trump occupies our conversation, but I have
chills and keep my coat on all through dinner. It's not a heavy
coat—I mean, it's spring—but it's a coat. I never say a thing about
being sick, much less about being married.

Louisa and Marie are loving and caring, and these two dinners
feel like betrayal. I mean, friendship betrayal. I take friendship
seriously. A friendship is a trust.

Then, also, there is my editor and the publicist at Blue Rider.

I feel as if I'm betraying them too. They are planning my *Siracusa* paperback tour and I want to cut it down. Flying from one city to another—I'm not physically and mentally up to it. I cancel the first part, which is the East Coast. My editor writes and asks me to please reconsider. I also cancel my trip to the UK for *Siracusa*'s British publication. I'm supposed to take part in festivals there. How can I cancel this book travel without explaining why?

This double life—I'm troubled by it. Many sick people keep their illnesses secret. There's no right or wrong. This decision is personal. It can't be judged. But that's a lonely place for me.

I plan to discuss it with Dr. Roboz.

She is already at the desk when I come into the clinic room. She explains my consolidation round—a second round of CPX, only two doses this time, not three. The purpose is to knock out any leftover malignant cells, called minimal residual disease. It's strange how information like this gets dropped. I had no idea I would have another round. Perhaps if I'd read about the treatment, I would have known. *Oh, a consolidation round? That's to secure the first-round results.* Okay. I will begin it as an outpatient on April 24, and when my white counts drop, ten to fourteen days later, I will be admitted to the hospital.

Then Dr. Roboz tells me that CPX is in the final stage of approval. The FDA, she says, can be capricious. It looks more favorably on new breast cancer drugs than on new leukemia drugs. Breast cancer seems to be the "cool" cancer, although she does not use that term. Would I write something about my experience? she asks. "We need patient advocacy for AML like there is for breast and prostate cancer."

I am so happy to do this. How often does one get to give back to a doctor? Being a patient is a passive place to live. If I write something, I can do my part for Dr. Roboz, for other patients with leukemia. I can, in a small way, contribute to the future of this life-saving drug. I will write a piece and hope to place it on the op-ed page of the *New York Times.*

I know instantly that having this article published is also my solution. I can reveal to everyone both my diagnosis and my marriage. I can tell all my friends and business associates at the same time, my way.

I am not my sister. At this moment, as I'm contemplating broadcasting my illness to the world in the newspaper, which is the last thing Nora would ever have done, this fact really hits home.

I have an idea how I want to write it. It starts cooking in my brain. "I thought I'd fallen into my own romantic comedy." That would be the lead.

I would begin the piece with the magic of meeting Peter (whom all my friends knew about), then I would proceed to reveal all the things that no one knew: my leukemia diagnosis, our wedding, this new drug CPX-351, my perilous hospital stay, Peter's constancy, fear and hope battling for my heart and mind. Finally, wondrously, remission.

I fuss like crazy over the piece. Jessie edits it patiently. Peter edits it. Deena edits it. Heather gives me notes. Dr. Roboz corrects all my medical facts. The *New York Times* accepts it.

Two nights before it is published, I send it to everyone: friends, family, business associates. I attach it to this group e-mail:

Group e-mail to everyone I know on May 26, 2017:

> Dearest family and friends:
>
> I need to tell you what's been going on with me. I am fine now, miraculously fine, writing, traveling (about to go on my paperback tour), but I have been sick and as a result out of touch and in some cases evasive and secretive. Please forgive me. I have written about what has been happening and, while it's a bit weird to do this, am sending it to you. It expresses my heart better than I could if I just wrote an email. Also I simply can't bear to call each of you directly. It would overwhelm me. The piece I've attached is running in the *New York Times* on Sunday, and I really don't want you to learn about me in the newspaper. Writing is how I make sense of everything. Please read it sitting down and forgive me for not being more direct. It's too difficult.
>
> All my love,
>
> Delia

The day that my *New York Times* piece is published in the Sunday Review section, my phone pings at 7:12 a.m. A text from Jon.

Am I missing your byline or was that intentional? he writes.

What? I text back. They left off my byline? R you serious?

I wake up Peter. "They left my byline off the piece," I tell him.

"What?" says Peter, sitting up in bed.

Needless to say, I was not expecting this. "My byline isn't on the piece." I'm sorry to keep repeating that, but I kept repeating it. That's not possible, except of course it absolutely is. I really, really can't compute it. We're at my brother-in-law's house and

I run downstairs to confirm it, to look at the newspaper on the kitchen table.

Obviously, the piece I sent to friends had my byline. It was a copy from my computer. And Peter had alerted his patients about the piece, summarizing it so that they didn't hear it first from the *Times*. But in the newspaper, on the actual printed paper, there is my piece with no name.

I have written maybe ten opinion pieces that have been published in the *New York Times,* and this has never happened. I read the Sunday Review section every week and, in my experience, every writer's name is always, always there. Nevertheless, I realize immediately that compared to being in remission, to being alive, this is a small disturbance. All day I am reminding myself that this is a comparatively small thing. Although it is the most intimate essay I have ever written, the most personal, and that is saying a lot because "personal" is what I do.

I e-mail my editor. She e-mails back. She is "mortified." She has no idea how this happened. My name is in the online edition, thank goodness, she says, and that's what most people read.

It's kind of a test. It feels like that to me. *Be grateful you're alive—this is nothing.* I do my absolute best not to obsess about it, not to complain, to let it go. And I do, sort of. Because I receive a flood of love. E-mails full of feeling—love, tears, and good wishes for my health and for my happiness with Peter. Marie writes, "Overjoyed... The coat should have told me." Joy calls it "scary and glorious news." Don: "Trembling." Bryan: "I just had a big cry." Joyce: "I cannot wait to meet this guy." Hope: "I love you." Lynn: "How brave and sad and wonderful." Aleks: "Your email triggered a cocktail of positivity in my two friends struggling to find their life love." Philip: "You are being well looked after by those in the next dimension." Diane: "I love you. I love Peter too. Please tell me his last name." Joe: "Peter is a giant." Meg: "Do you agree with me that Gail Roboz, whom I looked up, looks like an Ephron?" Patty: "Oh, oh, oh. There are too many plot points in this story." Kenny: "Really, miracle does not seem too strong a word." Everyone wants to meet Peter.

Through my website I receive not only good wishes from strangers but also their stories—about the joy of love late in life, about loss and heartbreak, about their own struggles with AML and other blood cancers, about giving them hope for new love and survival. A researcher studying ovarian cancer says my story encourages her to work harder.

To get this joy from friends and strangers is transporting. All this kindness. All this connection. It's like my feet leave the ground. Like I'm carried around on helium. It's also a bit scary, declaring my illness and health to the world. Remission isn't cure. Am I tempting fate? I repress those worries. Having this piece published is simply, magically, wonderful and, like a jackpot strike, for a very short time, it makes me feel invulnerable.

The piece hits number one on the *New York Times* most-e-mailed list. A friend sitting in a restaurant hears two diners talking about it. Someone else hears people discussing it on a SoHo street corner. My happiness is everywhere.

From Dr. Roboz to me:

Wow #1!!!!! I've heard from several people at the company, they are thrilled. They rarely get to know about individual patients and a happy story in the NYT is just huge.

CPX-351 was developed by a Canadian company called Cela-tor. During this final stage of approval, Celator sold the drug to Jazz Pharmaceuticals. Two days after my piece appears I receive this e-mail.

From Melody Nelson:

> Dear Ms. Ephron,
>
> I read your article about your journey with AML and your treatment with CPX-351. I remember the day my colleagues and I sat around a boardroom table in Vancouver wondering if our team could make that drug. It was 3rd on a list of about 8 potential drug combinations for different cancers. A lot of blood, sweat and tears followed over the past 15 years but we are grateful we're finally nearing the finishing line. I hesitated writing you but I felt compelled to let you know that the scientists who created and codeveloped CPX-351, I'm blessed to call them my friends, are amazing and wonderful human beings. Not just brilliant and hardworking but kind, generous, funny and compassionate. It's been a drug not created by "Big Pharma" (*sic*) which unfortunately has the reputation of being cold, callous, and money-hungry. It was a drug cultivated carefully by a small dedicated crew who wanted to help make a difference in the fight against cancer. I cry routinely lately thinking that it's actually happening but we never hear from patients. There's confidentiality of course so we don't know who they are. So your article touched me so deeply. Thank you for sharing it. Thank you for encouraging the FDA to move this along—we all agree, like you, that more people will need this. More people will undoubtedly respond like

you to CPX-351. Thank you for being brave and trusting in our drug during this clinical trial. I wish you many years of a happy, healthy life with your family.

    With deepest sincerity,

    Melody

This note is personal. So specific. A direct connection to the scientists and doctors who saved me. It makes them real. By writing this article, I've been able to thank them.

The impact of my *Times* piece on me, wonderful as it is, is short-lived. I am relieved at first because I don't have to keep up the pretense, but shortly after I am beset with worries again.

I have another bone marrow biopsy. "Fewer bad cells than last time," Dr. Roboz writes. I didn't realize I had any bad cells. My relationship to my illness is full of gaps in understanding. I thought my marrow was clear of disease. I have asked Dr. Roboz not to tell me too much, and I don't ask her to explain, and she doesn't. As a result, I am not really aware of what's going on. Except I get more and more anxious. And if I did know the details, the science of what my body is up to, I am sure it would not decrease my anxiety. My ability to spin things bigger is a scary talent. I figure Peter knows what's happening.

She prescribes an oral chemotherapy drug called Rydapt just before I leave for California for my paperback tour.

Me to Dr. Roboz, June 6, 2017:

> Subject: Rydapt
>
> After the pharmacy called yesterday to schedule a delivery for today and the drug didn't arrive, I called them and they said there was no delivery scheduled.
>
> I got hysterical crying (I am so frightened underneath it all) and now it's supposedly scheduled for tomorrow morning (wonderful Evgeny is double-checking on it) but I am panicked because it might not arrive before I leave tomorrow afternoon. I realized I don't even know if you want me to take it while I'm on the trip, or, if so, how much and, if it doesn't get here, if I'll die 'cause those chromosomes will mutate.
>
> Delia

All my e-mails about whether this drug will arrive and when to take this drug are like this. And what chromosomes am I even talking about? I don't think Dr. Roboz has ever mentioned chromosomes. All Dr. Roboz's return e-mails are calming.

Rydapt arrives the morning I leave for my book tour. I pack it, give Honey a hug, and leave her in the care of Lauren, our dog walker.

When I arrive in Northern California at the start of my tour, I am, well, *meshuga* (a Yiddish word meaning "nuts"). I manage to keep it mostly to myself, although I am beset with anxiety when we visit Peter's son. Naftali lives in the San Rafael hills and there are about twenty-three wooden steps down to enter his house. I am sure I will tumble down them. I worry that Idra, a sparkly two-year-old, will give me a cold and kill me when she dances around the room. How do I stay far enough away from her in the small living room? How do I get to know Peter's family under those circumstances?

I believe this is when I meet his daughter, Melina, and her partner, Matt, who live in Oakland. Melina, pregnant, has long ink-black hair, a wide smile, pale skin, deep red lipstick, and many tattoos. She looks like a beautiful punk princess. They are Northern California people—politically left and vegan. She is immensely smart, as is Matt (who will shortly be elected president of the Berkeley Teachers union). There is stuff I'm not used to, like taking off my shoes to enter their house (everyone in Peter's Bay Area world seems to take their shoes off inside), but it's all minor; they could not be nicer.

I visit bookstores in and around San Francisco. I celebrate Meredith's birthday, meet all her friends at a little party around an outdoor curvy swimming pool. There is a photo of me, Meredith, and her birthday cake. We are smiling. It is a lovely evening. I can be happy for short stretches when my internal panic is temporarily distracted. I fly to LA and give a talk at the Beverly Hills Public Library, which goes just fine except that they got my autobiographical information off my website, which I had not updated since Jerry died. The woman who introduces me says that I am married to the writer Jerome Kass and have a dog named Honey. Standing at the podium, I get hit with a wave of grief and have to take a minute to collect myself. They give me a present for Honey, a stuffed toy.

Afterward I have dinner with Phil and Jill. A lovely evening on their deck. Alex is there too, with his wife, Hope. Phil and Alex were both Jerry's students, and Alex met Hope because she was my niece's best friend and I took her to a party at my friend-daughter Heather's. Our worlds are all scrambled up in a great way. *Good family* is how I think of them, by which I mean friends that make you feel loved and safe.

During that evening in LA, my phone rings. It's Lauren, my dog sitter. "Something is wrong with Honey," she says. "She's listless. Something is very wrong." I tell her to take Honey to the twenty-four-hour emergency vet on Fifteenth Street and Fifth Avenue.

I hang up. I'm off to the side, speaking privately. Everyone at the dinner is eating. "Something's wrong with Honey," I tell them. They all know Honey.

Honey, thirteen years old now, has had cancer. In fact, she got her diagnosis in 2014 on the same day that Jerry and I learned that his prostate cancer was back. The day he learned he was no longer in remission, the vet phoned to say Honey had liver cancer. Honey had surgery and went into remission, but Jerry's remission was over. Dog cancer, people cancer, my cancer.

I'm feeling like a weak bird battling headwinds. A half hour later Lauren calls again. Honey's cancer is back. Viciously. She is dying. I speak to the vet. She will die shortly, she says, within twenty-four hours.

I am now absolutely without a mind. I can't make it work. Phil phones an airline and tells me there is one seat left on a red-eye. I am too scared to go. I am simply too frightened to go alone to the airport this night and get on a plane. I have no explanation for it and no excuse. Death is waiting for me there. I don't want to say that to them, I don't even want to admit it to myself. But there it is. I call Peter. He says he'll drive the six hours down to LA and pick me up tonight. I think . . . I can't think . . . it makes no sense. I start to obsess about my laptop, which is in San Rafael. How can I go back to New York without it? But really, it's not that. Fear has taken me over—my cancer, Jerry's cancer, Honey's cancer. They are all mixed up together.

I call the vet back. "Will she last two days?" I ask. She doesn't know.

If Peter drives down and picks me up and I get my computer in San Rafael, I can get back to New York City. I can say goodbye to her. I need my computer. This makes no sense. Peter could bring my computer tonight.

I don't believe anyone on this deck at this dinner knows my chaotic state. I am acting practical, and they are impressed that Peter is coming to get me. They are not dog people. No one here has a dog, although they love me and they know how much I love Honey. No one knows about the collision of my state of terror about my own remission with Honey's impending death. Or that, in my mind, Honey, Jerry, and I were a tribe.

I plead with the vet to try to keep her alive for two days. Lauren, who has walked Honey since she was a puppy, is with her. I console myself with that, but really, I am beating up on myself. It's no big deal to go to the airport and get on a plane. But I simply can't.

Peter arrives at one a.m. By seven or so we are on our way back north. My plan—now that Peter is with me and I am thinking more clearly, and he is comforting, always comforting—is to fly out on a red-eye tonight. But when we reach San Jose, Lauren calls again. Honey is not going to make it to tomorrow. The kindness would be to put her down now.

I explode in tears.

If you've ever lost a dog, you know it's a wipeout. But add to that my feeling that I've abandoned her, all that guilt and misery, her ties to Jerry, my own fragile state on this earth. That's a lot of combustion. But even without all that, dogs dig deep into your heart. They're in the room, on the floor, in your lap, on the bed, pestering you for treats, chewing your sock, burrowing under sheets, making you laugh, following you about, eating the cheese you left on the table, tearing in wild happy circles after baths. They trust. They are innocence. They are unjudgmental observers of your every unguarded moment.

The vet suggests that I visit with Honey on FaceTime so I can be with her when she euthanizes her. I am astonished and grateful she thinks of that.

About an hour later, as soon as we get to our apartment, I call. Lauren cuddles Honey so I can see her. She is a beautiful bundle of dirty white fur with big black eyes. I sing songs to her. They are ridiculous. I made them up and have sung them to her since she was a puppy. Lauren says that she can tell that Honey hears my voice. I don't know—can she? She can't smell me, she is frail, but she is looking into the phone toward me. I don't see the doctor or the needle, but suddenly her eyes dull and she is limp.

Now I am sobbing, absolutely unhinged.

Memories of Honey, they are all small and emotional. Daily bits of joy. Sometimes after a walk, Lauren would rinse her in the bathtub and I would come home and Honey would pop up over the side of the tub, struggling to get out to greet me. She would refuse to turn left when we exited the building because the dog washer was located in that direction—at least I think that's why she refused. When Fia, Phil and Jill's daughter, was about three, she and Honey would bark at each other, lying on their tummies on the living-room floor. Once Honey dug into my tote, found a chocolate cupcake, and ate it, carton and all. Then, since chocolate is poison to dogs, she had to have her stomach pumped. She was cheerful afterward. Actually, she was cheerful before too. I have photos of Jerry and Honey napping together on the bed. She was an easy dog, sweet. While at my desk writing, she would sit next to me and fix me with a stare: *I want a treat.* Sometimes she would just sleep by my feet. She got me through that first year after Jerry died.

Her complete name: Honey Pansy Cornflower Bernice Mambo Kass. Jerry named her Honey; pansy is my favorite flower; we passed a field of cornflowers bringing her home; Bernice is one of Jerry's favorite aunts; mambo is a great dance and a great word; Kass was Jerry's last name.

Honey—my last link to Jerry and our life together.

Me to Dr. Roboz, June 17, 2017:

> My legs are intermittently weak again. I'm being really careful and staying hydrated, which seems huge. Flying back tomorrow. My beloved dog died yesterday in NYC (I am in SF), unexpectedly suddenly very ill and I have been crying and upset for the last three days.

Dr. Roboz to me, June 17, 2017:

> Oh no Delia I am so sorry! How terrible! As a huge dog person who sobbed for weeks after I lost mine, I so understand the pain. I'm much more concerned about you mentally than physically at the moment, but full check-up coming soon. Don't let Peter stop hugging you. G.

At the end of June 2017 Peter shuts down his offices in San Francisco and Mill Valley. About half his patients continue on Zoom or phone. For the ones who want to move on, he makes sure they are safely settled. I continue this balancing act of new chemotherapy drugs to keep me in remission.

August 3, 2017:
The FDA approves CPX-351. It gets a name: Vyxeos.

Drug names are ridiculous. Giant amounts of consonants. Like they are all made up in Sweden. Or scientists throw a bunch of letters at a wall and see what sticks. But the letters in this case have meanings. *VI*—which, I'm told, they changed for aesthetic reasons to *Vy* (see how mysterious it all is?)—stands for the 5:1 ratio of the two drugs it contains, daunorubicin and cytarabine (those names are insane too). The *x* indicates a fixed ratio. *Eos* is the Greek goddess of dawn. *Os* is a reference to "overall survival," how long you will live after diagnosis with this drug.

The Greek goddess of dawn. How lovely she is tucked inside this crazy word.

The solar eclipse, coming soon, grips the country. There is a run on special glasses to protect our eyes from ultraviolet rays and allow us to look at the sun safely while the moon begins to obliterate it.

The eclipse will be visible to everyone in the continental United States on August 21, but to view the total solar eclipse, you have to be in the right location. Totality is everything, Peter tells me. Anything less doesn't cut it.

He made a reservation, long before we met, on Wallowa Lake in eastern Oregon. Wallowa Lake is not in the path of totality, but it is about two hours from Baker City, which is in totality. Eastern Oregon is desert, which is why Peter selected it. The possibility that there will be clouds obscuring nature's miracle is minimal.

Dr. Roboz is not thrilled about this trip. My white counts are low, but she decides they are safe enough, and she consents.

Peter has been to eastern Oregon. Years before he spoke at a NOMAS conference—National Organization for Men Against Sexism (his life is a history of being on the side of women; it always gives me shivers when he tells me this stuff)—at Lewis and Clark College in Portland. "Women, Men, Visions of Justice" was his subject. He spoke about sexual boundaries, sexual harassment. "Me being me," he said, "I drove there from San Francisco up through the Oregon desert and then down through the Columbia River Gorge." There he stopped at Multnomah Falls and stood on the lacy bridge hung between two cliffs that provides a head-on view of this six-hundred-foot cascade of water. "Like an eclipse," he said, "the falls are an unruinable bit of nature." He stayed for a night at the Eagle Cap Chalets, little one-room cabins in a pine forest on Wallowa Lake. That's where he booked for this phenomenon.

Here's what is amazing to me. The moon is 2,159 miles in diameter and has no light of its own. The sun is 864,938 miles in diameter and its radiance lights the world. For ninety seconds, because of the alignment of the sun, the moon, and Earth, this little moon takes over. It shuts out the sun.

To me, a solar eclipse is an underdog story. The all-time underdog event. A triumph of the small and weak over the giant and mighty.

A seemingly impossible feat.

I didn't know any of this before I met Peter, for whom the sky is a continual interest and enchantment, or before this coming eclipse fascinated everyone. I've enjoyed a lovely moon, but I've never followed wonderful crazy stuff like comets or eclipses. I have never seen the conjunction of Jupiter and Saturn. I cannot identify the Milky Way or Orion.

I love that the magic of the sky is coming into my life.

In Oregon, the eclipse will start at 9:05 in the morning. While the Earth rotates, bringing the moon and sun into alignment, we will all wear our special glasses, but at totality, 10:16 a.m., we take them off. Because at that moment it is safe to stare right at the sun.

We fly to Spokane, Washington, spend a night at a Ramada Inn, and then drive into the mountains to Wallowa Lake, where there's a small vacation town, some summer houses, and a lodge. Everything is low-key; nearly everything is made of logs. August is high vacation season, plus there is an eclipse, so the town is packed with visitors, hikers, and some park rangers with whom Peter chats about whether there will be traffic heading to Baker City tomorrow—they have no idea—and are they going? No, they are happy to see 98 percent totality here.

The next morning we're up at six to drive to Baker City, population a little under ten thousand. The roads are fairly clear, the two-lane Route 82 to Interstate 84. We bring potato chips because I never go anywhere without snacks. Baker City is at the northwest end of the Great Basin, a desert that stretches all the way into Utah. Our vistas are different now, no tall pines, mostly flat plains. We pull off the interstate and circle around a grassy lawn in front of a McDonald's. It's crowded with people on blankets awaiting totality.

This isn't where we want to see the eclipse, says Peter. It isn't suited to this epic event. We have to find a park or a field. We need a vista. We drive up and down residential streets worrying; will we find our ideal location in time? Finally, in the distance, Peter spots football stands. Baker High. Next to the football field is a worn grassy meadow. Bathrooms too. The view across the meadow to low hills is perfect.

Many people know this spot. There are small tents here and there. A group of Christian campers (ten- and eleven-year-olds) with their counselors pass the time singing folk-rocky Christian songs (sweet although we don't sit too close). A few people have set up cameras on tripods; there are families, couples, some solo guys in cowboy hats. Everyone sits on folding chairs or blankets. The air is still. It's not crowded or noisy. Nobody strikes up a conversation. No one is selling a souvenir. It's all respectful. People keep to themselves, spaced some distance apart. We're all here to see the moon do its thing.

Peter and I find our spot, sit on our parkas, put on our glasses, and wait.

I love these glasses. They are ridiculous-looking. Big cardboard frames printed with bits of yellow and orange planets and, over the bridge, the white glow of an eclipse. The lenses are black. Everyone staring upward wears some version of these. It's like we all belong to a cult.

Shortly after nine a.m. it begins. When I look at the sun, there is a tiny sliver of black, like a slice of pie, out of the sun's orb. It is clear. Definite. Startling.

It's riveting to look through these glasses and watch the moon eat up the sun. Over the next hour, this slice grows larger and larger, obliterating the sun more and more. During this time, when we lift the glasses, we see the world around us start to dull. The brightness is sucked out of the grass, color is drained from the hills, the sky's blue fades.

All the watchers are quiet. The effect is hypnotic.

Finally it's dark out, night at ten in the morning. Now we take off the glasses and see in the sky a black orb with a beautiful puffy white glow around it. Totality. Everyone applauds and cheers. It's a stunning show and what an achievement for a little moon.

There are few things we can experience the way people did thousands of years before us. Yes, the sun rises and sets, flowers bloom, seasons come and go, there is taste and smell. But this happened, too, before people understood astronomy. One day, they noticed dullness around them, watched as night fell when it should have been day. What was happening? It must have been terrifying. And then, ninety seconds later, the world began to light up again. A miracle.

It feels personal, although I'm embarrassed to compare my experience to this astonishing event. Is that underdog moon a metaphor of me versus the mighty leukemia?

Being faced with possibly fatal cancer has made me grateful for the love in my life, but it has not made me spiritual or religious. Still, I do feel that I was thrust into darkness and given back light. And it opened me up to feeling part of a larger world, I'm not sure why. Maybe because, in spite of being given a reprieve, it makes dying real. Like everyone else, I have a time here and it will be over.

Peter says some very early cultures, like the Mesopotamians in 4000 BC, saw eclipses as omens, and the Egyptians had some understanding of how they happened, but most of the ancient world was like me, earthbound and ignorant.

We drive from the eclipse straight back to Spokane. For lunch, we find a restaurant with truly delicious tacos, making this trip more perfect than ever. We spend the night at Northern Quest Hotel and Casino.

After we check in, Peter goes upstairs to our room and I go into the casino.

Jerry loved video poker. In the last years of his life, when he wasn't strong, we went to the Wynn in Las Vegas and played video poker for a few days. We never needed to leave the hotel. There were several restaurants, a spa, and exceptionally nice sheets on the bed (I bought some at the hotel store for our apartment). Sometimes we drove with friends to the somewhat tacky Resorts

World Casino on Rockaway Boulevard in Queens, where Jerry could blot out his illness and his worries. Video poker is basically throwing money away, but at twenty-five cents a play, it is mindless and fun.

I don't think Peter would ever go near a video-poker machine—he doesn't have a gambling bone in his body. I guess I go into the Spokane casino because casinos were places Jerry and I had happy times. It's crowded, messy, and noisy, full of people and slot machines crammed together. I wander around, feeling uncomfortable, hunting for some twenty-five-cent poker machines.

I stop for a minute, considering whether to stay or leave, and I hear Jerry say, *Delia*. I hear it absolutely. His voice floats in the air. He's calling me. He is not exactly next to me, but he's nearby.

I look every which way. I peek around in the vicinity. I walk here, walk there. I find only strangers playing slots. Confused, I assure myself, *I heard that. I heard that!* I go up to the room.

"I just heard Jerry's voice in the casino," I tell Peter. "He called my name."

Peter nods.

I guess after years of listening to patients' tales of their lives, nothing surprises him. "What *was* that?" I say.

"Hearing the voice of your dead spouse is normal and not unusual. You liked being in casinos together, right?"

"Okay, Doctor. But what was that? Was it him? I heard it, I absolutely heard it."

Peter shakes his head. "I don't know what it is. I only know it's normal."

Normal? Was it normal when Jerry and Nora were sick for me to go to North Carolina and find things I had already written in the novel that got me through those difficult days? Maybe Jerry is saying, *Hi. This casino—this is our place.* Maybe Jerry knows Honey is dead. That's magical thinking, right? But hearing Jerry's voice was magical. So perhaps he's comforting me. Maybe he knows that when I get back to New York City and open the front door, I won't hear Honey's paws racketing up the stairs. And he's saying to me, *We're still here.*

As soon as we get back from Oregon, I'm at the hospital for three days of decitabine infusion taken in conjunction with Rydapt—two pills a day, one every twelve hours. I am religious about Rydapt, anxious that if I'm off the mark, it won't work. These pills are the size of submarines. I remember dropping one down my throat without water on the corner of Union Square West and Seventeenth Street.

So chemotherapy continues. I'm in remission but these additional drugs are working to keep me there. There is ugly stuff in the world, like Harvey Weinstein's abuses of women. The #MeToo movement is both depressing and encouraging. I wonder how much work I haven't been offered because I'm female, something I never fixated on. Although I have thought often about how much the movie business is controlled by men and the interests of men. It is simply a given. Working with Nora, which was what I mostly did, protected me because she was a director and she was tough. At the same time, I understood that I needed to have my own voice as a writer. I had my own stories to tell. That meant I needed to write books. I'm glad I don't have regrets about how I shaped my writing life, always trying to mix it up, novels, nonfiction, screenplays. I was lucky that I could switch. In empty moments, trying not to think about where this illness is going, I sort of evaluate my past. I'm relieved that my choices make sense in retrospect.

I've gotten to make my living by my imagination. That's a lovely thing.

The eclipse has pepped me up. The magic of it. The adventure—sitting in a high-school field watching the world disappear and re-appear. I am beginning to believe with absolutely no evidence at all that my remission will be a long one or at the very least will last a full fourteen months, until next summer.

Peter and I, feeling optimistic and festive, plan a party to celebrate our union. We send an e-vite with a photo of us in our eclipse glasses, gazing upward, awaiting totality.

To celebrate our marriage
Please join us for cake, champagne, and Ping Pong
Sunday, October 29th
2 to 5 p.m.

Eugene bakes a spectacular tiered cake, half chocolate, half yellow, covered in white roses with sugar markers of our love story, including the record "Come in Stranger," Peter's Subaru, the Grand Canyon, and the eclipse. It's pouring rain that day, but I don't take it personally. I'm so happy. I set up two Ping-Pong tournaments, one for more experienced players (people who can hit slams, for instance; I ask them to evaluate themselves). Our apartment fills with friends. Alice—Peter's friend, who is rapidly becoming mine too—sews us a pot holder with the photo of us gazing at the eclipse printed on the fabric. Every time I use it to pick up a hot pot, I will think of that happy moment.

We are full of plans. For Thanksgiving, we will go to Paris, then fly to Wales so Peter can meet Richard and Julia. Then at Christmas, we will fly back to San Francisco to see Peter's family.

In Paris we stay at a cozy Left Bank hotel where the bed takes up most of the room and do simple things: stroll around, sip coffee and wine for hours in cafés watching Parisians go by, visit an outdoor market where we buy a roast chicken that we rip apart and eat on a nearby bench. We visit favorite places, like the Luxembourg Gardens, and do a pastry walk. A pastry walk is a long walk—my favorite is through the sixth arrondissement, then along Rue de Bayonne in the seventh—and at every bakery we pass, we go in and buy every single thing that looks remotely tasty: apple turnovers, croissants, pain aux raisins, eclairs, almond things, chocolate concoctions, cookies, anything lemon. Then, loaded down with these rapturous goods, we return to the hotel, order tea or coffee, and taste them all.

I have a photo of Peter smiling his electric smile on the Pont Notre-Dame, and another I like even more on the same bridge: his eyes are closed, his lips together but breaking toward laughter. It's like he's having the most wonderful dream. Looming behind is Notre-Dame—the Gothic masterpiece with its flying buttresses and giant circular rose windows that look as delicate as snowflakes.

The beauty of Paris is reassuring, its constancy. I'm grateful for places that haven't changed, because I have. (A year and a half later, Notre-Dame will burn.)

Before flying to Birmingham and taking a taxi across the Welsh border to the Wye Valley, I have a worried exchange with Dr. Roboz because Richard and Julia's grandson had chicken pox when he visited their house the week before. We are all concerned that some germs stayed in the air and I can catch it. Is this paranoid or is it reasonable? I have no idea. Dr. Roboz never acts as if my questions are neurotic or panicky. I am cleared to visit.

When we land, Howard, the local taxi driver, picks us up. He always picks me up, whether I'm in Birmingham, Bristol, or Heathrow. There is a coziness to this Welsh world. On one of my last visits before Jerry died, I left my wallet containing all my dollars and pounds on the bar in a restaurant in Monmouth, Julia and Richard's nearest town, which is several quaint blocks. I didn't know I'd left my wallet in the restaurant. I could have left it at the church where we went to a crafts earring sale or the hardware store where I bought a plug adapter or somewhere else, like under the car seat. I only knew I'd lost it and I was quite agitated.

The phone rang at Richard and Julia's house at ten that night. It was a policeman, who said this: "The constable on the hill"—I have no idea who this was and I don't believe Richard or Julia did either—"said that the Gregsons have a visitor from America and perhaps this wallet is hers." Well, it was, and he delivered it the next day to their front door, all the money inside.

The Wye Valley is a whimsical place located at the intersection of eccentricity and beauty. The hills are a lush plush green, speckled here and there with old farmhouses and towering trees and, in the spring, carpets of bluebells. Sheep and cows poke their heads over the low stone walls. Julia has a few chickens meandering around, which means fresh eggs. There are tennis courts somewhere (I've never seen them) that everyone plays on all year. Sometimes it's so foggy Julia can't see her opponent. When Poppy got married— Poppy is Richard and Julia's daughter—she had a cake out of a storybook. Baked by Tori, a local baker, it was about twenty thin layers of sponge with strawberry cream in between. It narrowed at the top like a mountain but tilted slightly on the way up, like an elf's cap. It looked like something out of *Alice in Wonderland*. Like the Mad Hatter was going to show up any second and give a toast.

Their house, an old farmhouse, is not big but it is crammed with cozy rooms. The windows are small and the views seem like little landscape paintings. Peter and I can't stay here because of Richard's Parkinson's disease. He has to sleep downstairs now in what I always considered to be my room. Parkinson's is a wicked illness, slowly diluting his ability to be in the world. His voice is faint, his gait unsteady, but he is, as always, charming, smart, and, most of all, interested in other people. Conversation flows way into the night, although sometimes Richard snoozes in the middle. He has been falling, and this house, which was mostly built in the eighteenth century but with origins as early as the thirteenth, has a narrow staircase with turns in it where one can easily lose one's balance or, if one doesn't remember to bend, crack one's head on the ceiling. (The bed-and-breakfast we stay at, about twenty minutes away, has stairs like this too. Treacherous. It must be a specialty in ancient Welsh architecture.) The kitchen, dining room, and living room are mixed up together in a snuggly way, always warmed by the fireplace and the Aga. Peter has never seen an Aga, this gigantic iron cooking invention. I get to explain to him how it works, that the ovens and circular metal iron-topped grills are always on. I show him that you switch a pan from a high-heat grill to a low-heat one and control the cooking that way. It's like knowing a foreign language.

We hang out for hours around the table, as I did before with Jerry, and it doesn't feel odd. Peter immediately likes Richard and Julia, who are welcoming and interested, and he is folded into the affection between us. This is the magic of their home. No one can resist the pull of love and conversation. Jelly takes a day to remember me and then is always nosing in for a pat.

Richard's walking is unsteady and slow. It takes him quite a while to get anywhere—from the front door to the car, from the heavy wood rectangular dining-room table to the small round bridge table. Julia has his pills on a timer, and every so often its bell goes off, startling us all, and Julia rushes to get the pills. God, illness is such an interference, and yet Richard's brain is as sharp as ever. He is still the best bridge player of the four of us and likely to make outrageous bids that turn out to be smart. I have my time alone with him when Julia and Peter go hiking. Richard still calls me "darling" in a heart-melting way. He tells me I'm brave to fall in love again and urges me on in my writing as he always does. Of course he approves of Peter; how could he not? Peter is easy in company—interested in other people, never needing center stage but always participating. And Peter has, everyone agrees, saved me. Richard tells me about his latest hospital adventure in a ward with sixty other patients. I am stunned by the number sixty, so stunned I fixate on it, and I don't even hear the funny stories he tells, making his painful surgery recovery sound like an adventure. He and Julia love the National Health Service, which provides free health care for every UK citizen. We discuss his daughter from a previous marriage, Natasha, a favorite topic. He always worries about her since she's in America and he's not. I assure him she's doing brilliantly. We don't discuss death. Not that we avoid it. It's just that here, we're preoccupied with life.

Richard and Julia live near the ruins of Tintern Abbey, a church built in the twelfth century and destroyed by Henry VIII in the sixteenth century when he broke with the Catholic Church. What's left are the stone bones: walls; arches supported by columns but no roof; empty domed spaces where once windows with intricate stained-glass filtered the light; grass where there should be floor. It's moving, the way it stands there decimated. I fear I might be identifying with it: standing but decimated. Not just me—me and

Richard. My ability to take amazing phenomena—eclipses, falling-down ancient churches—and relate them to myself is overblown and nearly preposterous but also evidence of how preoccupied I am with my fragile state. We take Peter to visit.

Julia loves poetry—well, we all do, but she knows more than the rest of us, and there is a book of Wordsworth's poems next to the fireplace. She and Peter recite, alternating lines, "Tintern Abbey" by Wordsworth, a poem about—very roughly, forgive me—how the poet's love of the Wye Valley, of nature, his memories of his childhood here, have kept him...well, to keep it simple, sane. The magical power of this place—we all feel it.

We leave with promises to return in the spring.

Delia to Julia and Richard, November 29, 2017:

Ohmygod, it was blissful and magical to be in Whitebrook. To introduce Peter to the bliss of your home, the conviviality, curiosity, love, affection, conversation ...all the joy which you both create. I was so happy. After last year and all we have been through together. And to find that Peter was a match for us three in a new and wonderful way. How divine. Julia, I can't believe you trekked us back and forth and I see in my head all the dishes I left you with. The mystery of the laundry, so happy to have my lace undies back.

Much excited about how much Peter loved you both and Wales and has already discovered a NYC one-stop Dublin to Bristol. Which he thinks is better. I love you both so much. Our friendship is truly one of the great things of my life.

All my love,
Delia

November 30, 2017

I have a bone marrow biopsy as soon as we return and get the results from Natalie, Dr. Roboz's PA.

Peter and I are sitting opposite her at the clinic table. Feeling good and positive and certain I am fine. Natalie says, "The results indicate early relapse."

"What?"

Natalie nods.

"The disease is back?"

"It's coming back. Yes."

"Where's Dr. Roboz?" I say.

Natalie looks nearly tragic. "She's at a conference. She's in Japan. Do you think *I* would be telling you this if she were here?"

part six

O to A

$\mathcal{P}$eter remembers it differently. And in more medical detail.

Natalie is able to tell us only that there are warnings of a recurrence. It isn't until two weeks later, when the cytogenetic results from the bone marrow biopsy come back—these results take much longer—that Dr. Roboz can see that the chemotherapy, effective in a temporary way, has not been able to change the abnormalities of my chromosomes. The cytogenetics—the scientific study of chromosomes, to put it simply—make it clear the leukemia is coming back.

"AML is like Whac-a-Mole," says Dr. Roboz when she sees us. "You knock it down in one place and it pops up in another."

"Are there other drugs for me?" I stand and move back. I need to get out of the room. I don't want to hear this.

"Yes," she says. "But I don't think they will work for long." I hear the toughness. I know from the way she says this that one day she will tell me it's over. She will do it because, nice and kind as she is, she's the doctor, it's her job. "Your recurrence is early, at only eight months." This even with the assistance of other chemotherapy drugs like Rydapt. She means my AML is fierce. "The only thing that will actually 'cure' AML is a bone marrow transplant."

"I don't have a match," I say. I believe this because Nora and I were matched six years ago, and, except for me, Nora didn't have one.

"I want you to meet Dr. Koen van Besien, director of our stem cell transplant program." She adds some other things, like how much I will like him. While sitting there, I remember Dr. Roboz once mentioned a post-transplant patient suffering from graft-versus-host disease who complained that he never should have let her talk him into this. It was an offhand remark at a time when my future with chemotherapy drugs was more optimistic.

Natalie walks in and hears Dr. Roboz mention the transplant. "It's a year of your life," says Natalie. "And then you are fine."

"I don't have a match," I tell her.

I repeat this to Peter several times a day and to anyone else I'm trying to keep updated on the progress of my illness. It isn't necessarily new information to them. It is more said to myself, spoken with dull flatness, pounding the dismal reality into my brain.

About having a match: There are organizations, the most well-known being Be the Match, where healthy people can sign up to provide their lifesaving stem cells to people who are dying of various blood diseases. Leukemia is one. After you register, you receive an envelope with instructions and three long Q-tips. You take three swabs—one from inside the left cheek, one from inside the right cheek, and one from inside the lower and upper lips. You mail them in. The organization analyzes your DNA for HLA markers. These are critical. HLA (human leukocyte antigen) markers are found in most cells in your body, and your immune system uses them to determine which cells belong in your body and which do not. The closer the patient's HLA matches the donor's HLA, the better. There are twelve points doctors look at in finding an HLA match. A twelve-point match is a perfect match.

You might register with Be the Match and never get a call to save someone's life. Or you might get a call a week later. Or ten years later. You might live in Portugal and be a match for someone in Canada. It's a worldwide registry and medical cooperating system. It's remarkable. If you are a match for a sick person, the organization will contact you. If you still want to participate, you will be given a physical, including a CBC (complete blood count), and you'll have your medical history reviewed. If all that checks out, you will go to a hospital that participates in the program. You will get hooked up to a machine that withdraws your blood, harvests your stem cells, and circulates your blood back in. It takes about five hours and it's painless. Blood stem cells are the immature cells from which most blood cells in your body develop. Those harvested stem cells are shipped to the patient's hospital and transfused into the sick patient.

At some time in the past several years, bone marrow transplants also became known as stem cell transplants. This is because the method of extracting the stem cells changed; they are no longer collected straight from the donor's marrow. The new procedure, now done by transfusion, is much easier on donors. The terms *stem cell transplant* and *bone marrow transplant* tend to be used interchangeably.

My "I don't have a match" meant that there was no perfect twelve-point HLA match for me in the system. I didn't understand the science then, and thank God, I didn't ask. Thank God, I had never heard of HLAs and how, if I got a stem cell transplant from a donor who wasn't a good match, they would be dancing around in my body attacking these new stem cells that could save my life.

December 20, 2017

The transplant clinic is located at the far end of the third floor. Exit the elevator, walk left for Dr. Roboz, right for Dr. van Besien (or "VB," as everyone calls him).

The small waiting room has a sign:

ATTENTION
In order to protect our
patients and staff,
ALL PATIENTS and anyone coming
in with flu symptoms are
required to wear a mask in this
area

Masks are required because transplant patients have severely compromised immune systems. In the cure, your marrow is emptied and your entire immune system vanishes, and until it builds up again— new red cells, new white cells, new platelets—you are at risk.

Because of my own vulnerability, I always wear masks now in the hospital but we take them off after we are escorted to clinic room 26. It's a plain, small room with two metal chairs where Peter and I sit side by side. In front of us is an examining table. Dr. van Besien comes in and shakes our hands. He sits on the side next to the computer. He's in his late fifties, I guess, tall, with deep-set eyes, thinning gray hair. He has a kind of quiet dignity. He also has an accent—of course he does, since he is Belgian—so there is a soft spin on his words, like he might be French, but not. In this meeting I understand what he's not more than what he is. He's not arrogant. Assured but not arrogant. I'm relieved about that.

We don't chat. There is no preliminary.

He describes the transplant. I will have a round of chemotherapy first to clean out the disease in my marrow. I don't know what this chemotherapy consists of, but I know from my sister, who researched it, that it is brutal. Then, if the chemotherapy is successful, I will get a transplant from two donors: one from the blood of an adult, one from the umbilical cord blood of a baby. Mothers can donate their cord blood when they give birth. This cord blood is immensely adaptable, which is helpful when the match isn't perfect, but there is not much of it. It will migrate to my empty marrow. While it takes root and begins to multiply, the adult donor will take care of me. Then the adult donor fades away.

Why does the adult donor mother the baby donor, then let it take over? It seems miraculous. Some science sounds like science fiction.

Dr. van Besien knows, I assume from Dr. Roboz, that it's likely I don't have a perfect match. That's why he's not proposing a single-donor bone marrow transplant but this newly emerging method—a transplant from two donors. It's called a haplo-cord transplant.

I do not understand on this day that this is a new, experimental transplant. I don't remember even hearing the term *haplo-cord transplant.* I don't know that this haplo-cord transplant was invented by doctors in Spain or that Dr. van Besien has worked on making it more effective. Or that few hospitals do it. That day I hear only certain things.

Dr. van Besien says the matches from both donors will be imperfect. How imperfect? I don't ask that. I don't say, *If I don't have a twelve-point HLA match, how many HLA points do my matches and I have in common?* I don't know anything about HLAs or twelve-point matches. I am both too ignorant to ask the question and too terrified. I don't have any idea how Dr. van Besien evaluates matches. The one thing I do understand is that this haplo-cord transplant is probably the only thing that can save my life.

My ignorance through this illness—my not wanting to know or understand the science or simply not being able to take it in, losing what is told to me, never investigating what is, leaving my Google absolutely unused—is not surprising to me. It isn't only that I know Peter, being a doctor, will sort it, because Peter's nature, new to me too, is not fully part of my understanding. When you're facing death, I think, character is still destiny. I am curious about many things and write about them—how people fall in love, why marriages break up, family madness, family dynamics, psychological cruelties, childhood, the nature of friendship—but about the science of saving my life, I know only this: If I do research I will panic, I will become hysterical, I will misunderstand, I will obsess. I don't even have an appetite for it. I'm not repressing curiosity. I simply trust my ability to choose people and then abdicate.

Here's what Dr. van Besien says at our first meeting that I do retain: "You are over seventy. Many hospitals won't attempt a bone marrow transplant on a person over seventy." You can't survive it is obviously the reason. He isn't mean, he speaks kindly, but he's not trying to get my business. "Go across the street," he suggests. "See what they say there." He means Sloan Kettering. I'm not going across the street. I'm not leaving Dr. Roboz. *We're on the Roboz train.* I don't tell him that.

"Your odds of this working are twenty percent," he tells me. My age, no perfect match, the existing disease in my marrow. Transplants work only if you can wipe the marrow clean first. "If you don't have a transplant," says Dr. van Besien, "you have four months, maybe four and a half months left."

How ordinary I feel sitting here in this little metal chair listening to someone give me the most awful news. I don't cry. I twitch a bit, squirm, but barely react.

"Peter and I just fell in love," I say.

I have no idea why this pops out. Some desire not to be just another patient who walks into his clinic room. Some notion that "love" might increase my odds or lengthen my time. Some reason to explain why I might do something as crazy as try a transplant with a 20 percent chance of survival.

"Think about it," he says. "Come back in a week."

That afternoon I bump into Gail (not Dr. Gail Roboz; another impressive Gail. I'll call her Gail M.) in the lobby of my building.

Gail M. is a psychotherapist. I have always wanted her to be my psychotherapist, although you really can't have a psychotherapist you bump into every time you walk your dog—although I no longer have a dog. She is walking her dog Moki.

Moki liked Honey and likes me, which is rare for Moki. He is a coton, a fluffy white pup about the same height as Honey but considerably wider and fatter and much more particular about people. Ever since I moved in, Gail M. and I have chatted on the street. Deeply and personally. That's our friendship—lobby and street. I confided in her when Jerry was sick. After Jerry died, she left delicious home-cooked meals for me with the doorman, vegetarian concoctions along with a baguette. She plays the banjo, although I have never heard her, but she is often off to banjo lessons. She's in her sixties, very alive, small, with short wavy hair, a yellow blond, and she often wears wild crazy prints. When I met Peter, I practically screamed when I bumped into her. "I can't believe it. And he's a shrink!" She told me how she met Marti, the woman she is married to. She was about to take final vows as a nun when she attended a seminar for psychiatric social workers Marti was teaching. She took one look at Marti, fell madly in love, and that was that.

I blurt it all out in the lobby: "It's back again, I'm out of remission." I beg her to come to my apartment.

We sit upstairs, me on the couch, she across in a wicker chair, beautiful afternoon light.

When I asked her about this meeting later, she described me as being "in utter and complete undefended terror." Terrified to start the process, terrified they wouldn't find a match, terrified to die. She told me my terror was so powerful, "I felt merged with that terror."

"If I do this," I ask her, "will you help me?"

Poor Gail M., lassoed by a crazed neighbor who has leukemia and roped in. She has, I think, the biggest heart. I know that. I take advantage of her heart. She says of course she'll help. She'll talk to me as much as I need before I get the transplant, she'll come to the hospital during. When I walk her to the elevator, I say, "It's very important that you love me."

Now, I have to say, I have no memory of saying this, but Gail M. told me later that I did and that it shocked her. It shocks me too. Bad enough I begged her to join me in this catastrophe, in this tragic, frightening attempt to circumvent death, but then I told her that she also had to love me. To me, this is a sign of how unhinged I was.

She thinks about it as the elevator doors open. "Well, Delia," she says, "it's not a problem because I do love you."

She told me later that she knew, at that moment, she was going to take this trip with me.

I was amassing my women warriors. Looking back now, even before I decided, I was assembling my troops.

Christmas Day—more of the same: Should I or shouldn't I? Extreme agitation. Maybe a walk on Tenth Street. In and out of Peter's office. He lets me rant. He thinks I should do it. He knew I would, he told me later, but he wanted me to find my own way there. I'm not into holidays. It sounds bleak, but it's burnout. Years of decorating, shopping, wrapping, baking cookies with sprinkles, baking Maida Heatter's mousse torte, Maida Heatter's coffee-toffee pie, a ham, having a big party every year on Christmas Day—it wore me out. Or maybe I'm just not into celebrating something I could describe as my last Christmas.

Slightly crazed, sometime between Christmas and New Year's, I totter over to Nix on University Place for lunch with Sarah, a screenwriter and novelist. We met picketing on the first day of the Writers Guild strike in 2008. By the time we'd circled the block a few times, we knew we were friends. I tell her the second I slide into the booth: "I'm sick again." Her face crumples. She sits there quietly taking it in. I tell her about the transplant, give her my odds, 20 percent, and tell her I might not do it. "But you're in love," she says. "I mean, you've just fallen in love."

$\mathcal{D}$r. Roboz phones to discuss it. I'm sitting on the bedroom couch, the same place I was sitting when she confirmed I had AML nine months ago. "Dr. van Besien says I have a twenty percent chance of its working, of my surviving," I tell her. "Twenty percent. That is nothing."

"You are not a statistic," she says.

This is the only possible response, right? I'm being cynical, but she seems to mean it. She spells it out—my healthy heart and lungs, good blood pressure, no diabetes, excellent liver and kidneys, and so on, all my assets not visible on the outside. In return, I lay out the awful things I have heard about the treatment: that the chemotherapy is brutal, the graft-versus-host disease debilitating, that it could kill me.

Dr. Roboz says, "Don't be scared of the treatment, be scared of leukemia."

That is, of course, it: Don't be scared of the treatment, be scared of leukemia. She changes the focus of my terror.

I decide pretty much at that moment I might as well go out fighting. For me and for Peter. I think of something else too. A long-ago memory. When a fertility doctor was trying to figure out why I couldn't have children, forty or so years ago, he told me about this one condition but said I probably didn't have it because it was rare. Only 10 percent of the women who can't have children have this condition, he said. It turned out I had it. So, you know, there are actual people who make up the small percentages. In the case of my bone marrow transplant, a positive small percentage. I could be one of the lucky 20 percent.

Out of this convoluted, mixed-up thinking, I manage to spin a little hope.

We have our second appointment with Dr. van Besien. In this meeting he stands up and says, "I think you should do it." He also ups my odds. They are now 40 percent.

I don't know why he ups my odds. It's not like he acknowledges he's upping them. He doesn't say, *I said twenty percent last time, but now I think it's forty.* He just says, "Your odds are forty percent." Is this some new assessment of my energy? My overall health? A more careful reading of my current bone marrow situation? Did Dr. Roboz ask him to up my odds? "I think you should do it." Was that him or Dr. Roboz?

I don't ask, *Why did you up my odds?* Peter doesn't either.

I believe doctors rarely have any idea how helpless patients can be when their brains are jumbled by fear, how unable they are to respond or take information in. Or maybe it's just me. I'm lame. Exceptionally lame. Of course, 40 percent is still low, and I don't believe it anyway. I'm just scared of leukemia. I would now rather go out this way.

December 27, 2017

I wake up remembering a woman I met at a book signing over a year ago. She sent me a note after my *New York Times* piece. I frantically comb through my e-mails.

To me from Elyse Martin:

> Hi Delia,
>
> I met you at your book talk in Lake Forest last year. I was the woman that was convinced we were related because I resemble your sister Nora and we're from the same town in Belarus. On ancestry I even have a cousin listed with the name Ephron. I just read your piece in the *New York Times* and wanted to tell you how happy I was that you found love at 72. That gives me hope! And that I am so relieved that you are in remission. What a year you've had. Thanks for sharing your story.
>
> Xo
>
> Your cousin (I think)
>
> Elyse Martin

Elyse did look like Nora. She looked more like Nora than I did. And Nora and I looked quite a lot alike. She is undoubtedly a relative. My God, maybe she is my match. I e-mail and ask if I can phone her. She says fine.

I am hopping around, hoping I have solved this. Hoping I can send my odds through the roof.

We talk. I explain that my leukemia is back and I need a match for a bone marrow transplant. I ask her if she would consider being typed. I tell her what little I understand about that and what it will mean if she's a match. Elyse instantly agrees. She could not be nicer or kinder.

I run it by Dr. Roboz, who says, point-blank, given my sister's and my both having AML, we must assume leukemia could run in the family. Leukemia can be inherited. She doesn't want to match me with anyone who has an Ephron gene.

Peter is tested. We imagine that somehow, with all the magic between us, maybe he's a match. He isn't.

I don't let the possibility of my "cousin" go and send a pleading e-mail to Drs. Roboz and van Besien: "I have a hunch she is at least a partial match." I also add new information that she has a cousin who died of leukemia and her father died of lymphoma. Dr. Roboz says, "I am not psyched for a family member, especially with this additional family history." But she defers to VB.

He says, "There are no risks to the typing...if she ever would be a donor—which I highly doubt—then there would be very, very small risk for complications."

While I am getting more anxious and more tired and developing sores from blood pooling inside my mouth under my skin—showing signs, I believe, of the return of leukemia—I send all VB's and Dr. Roboz's e-mails to Meredith, my genius medical friend, to sort out for me.

"Given the way your mind works," writes Meredith, "you'd get focused on the risk. I'd let it go. Believe the magic will come from another source or thing!"

I move on from Elyse. I am now in van Besien's hands. Trust. This is a big thing: I am handing my life over to this doctor, and only Peter will be looking out for me. It's a game I cannot win on my own. I have never before felt utterly helpless.

The hospital sends endless information about the transplant. I will be in the hospital at least six weeks, then in a hotel next door to the hospital for outpatient supervision every day for a while, then home. Assuming it works. My ultimate recovery will take almost a year. During this time, there are many, many rules: No restaurants, no parties, no going to a theater, no subways or buses, no children, no babies, no dogs, no down pillows, no flowers, no strawberries, no grapes, no sushi, no delicatessen food (nothing sliced behind a counter), nothing premade that is sitting out there, like anything at a salad bar or a selection of chic cheese, no fruit without skin. Wash an orange or avocado before I cut and peel it. Wash the knife before I use it. One germ can wreak havoc.

Don't be scared of the treatment, be scared of leukemia. I keep Roboz's words in my heart as I tell friends about my pending transplant in sad phone calls and e-mails. Trying to organize. Peter will live in the hospital room with me. Linda will come afternoons in the hospital to spell him. Julia will fly in from Wales for a week. Deena will fly in from California when Peter's daughter has her baby so he can fly west to visit her. Jessie and Gail M. will visit when possible. I don't ask Meredith, as comforting and medically brilliant as she is, to come in from San Francisco because she has had her own medical traumas in the past and I don't want to burden her. As for my friend-daughters . . . Natasha will arrive at some point later. Jill too. Heather cannot because she has a baby. My nieces Anna and Rachel will visit early. Lisa, who was there for me the day Jerry died, can't come because she has a long-planned trip to India. My sisters offer to help.

Peter keeps everyone up-to-date by e-mail. And in the middle of all this, he decides he should retire. Giving his patients lots of time to adjust, he tells them in January 2018 that he will retire at the end of December.

To qualify for the transplant, I have to pass many tests, most in the same morning: bone density, blood tests, CT scan, echocardiogram, pulmonary function test, MRI. I must meet with the hospital social worker. I have to visit my dentist. He writes a note attesting that my mouth is trouble-free. Also I see my skin doctor, certain I have misbehaving moles. Which I don't. My anxiety is spreading, my panics abound, but actually, once you have had chemotherapy, your skin does become a dangerous place.

Sometime in here, my first adult donor is rejected. No one tells me why. "It often happens," says VB.

Most important, Drs. VB and Roboz put me in another clinical trial for CPX-351 (I don't think I'll ever get used to calling it Vyxeos). This trial is to test the drug's effectiveness as a chemo-therapy before transplants.

I still have leukemia in my marrow, and for this transplant to work, I need to be fully in remission. Roboz and VB don't want to trust this to the regular transplant chemo. I will have that too, of course, but I will start with a round of CPX.

CPX has to work its magic again. My future is in its hands. If the marrow isn't wiped clean, the doctors won't proceed. I sign the papers to be in the trial.

Thursday, January 25, 2018

I have a tunneled catheter installed at interventional radiology. It's just below my collarbone and to the right. It's like a port but with another name. Now I have a built-in door for all daily blood draws, transfusions, and chemotherapy.

Tuesday, January 30, 2018

The new adult donor comes through.

Wednesday, January 31, 2018

Peter hears that the hospital will arrange "protected private space" for him to conduct phone or video sessions with his patients. I'm not the only soul in his trust.

Saturday, February 3, 2018

Eugene chops off my hair, all but the tiniest shag. I love my hair. It's thick and a bit too curly, but as I've gotten older, accepting all sorts of diminishments, wrinkles, and flab, there's always been my legs and my hair. I could count on them. I'm down to my legs now. I don't let myself feel this loss. I just do it. I mean, what's the point compared to everything else?

Eugene and I don't talk about this momentous thing. Although he spins the chair away from the mirror. Instead we discuss my wig. He has a friend, Luc, who is brilliant at wigs, and Luc and Eugene will come to the hospital for a fitting. I'm like a soldier, doing what I'm ordered to, no choice. Trying to feel nothing. Also, I don't want to mourn. I'm looking ahead—what do I need, not what will I lose.

Don't be scared of the treatment, be scared of leukemia.

Sunday, February 4, 2018

I pack for six weeks in the hospital, from which I may never return. My sister Amy sends cute pajamas; Julia sends a silk kimono-like robe. From a drawer, I retrieve all the sweats and T-shirts Mitch, my beloved neighbor, has gifted. Natasha, at my request, sends me a mountainous assortment of moisturizing lotions.

Monday, February 5, 2018

*P*eter fills out the forms in the admission office, and I am in.

I get a couple of days on the fancy floor, have my first CPX infusion here. I keep checking for a single room on the oncology wing because I will have to move there when CPX hopefully begins to work its magic.

By now I have spent so much time (including getting married) in this lovely wing with its free waffle-weave robe and river view, I'm beginning to think of it as a place where I have a time-share. Like on an island. Since I may or may not survive this, I am not trying to save money. Two days here, then a single room on the oncology wing. Drain my account, it's fine with me.

The transplant wing, Ten West, is all single rooms because the patients have very low immunity. Visitors have to wear masks. I will land there only if CPX puts me in remission.

On the first day, the oncologist making rounds stops in. I'll call this person Dr. C. (That's not the doctor's real initial.) Dr. C. sits down in my room and says, unasked: "You might be immune to CPX."

Immune? I had no idea I could develop immunity to my lifesaving drug. If I'm immune, I'm screwed. Instantly my fragile hopes plummet. Instantly I am furious. Instantly I hate this doctor.

Yes, hate.

I am for sure full of rage right now, although giving the impression, I believe, of being merely anxious. But looking at an endgame—going to endless tests, trying to trust bleak odds, talking and thinking about the mess of me every single second—of course I'm also angry. Scared too. And looking for someone to dump it all on. When Dr. C. tells me it could all be over soon, that I could be immune, this doctor is it. I've found my target.

Patient at risk for adverse outcome from underlying disease and chemotherapy treatment. Dr. C. inserts that note in my record (I discovered later) after every visit. Just to remind everyone that I might not make it, and if I ever do get into danger, of course this brilliant doctor knew it all along. And nurses can dismiss any catastrophe with *Wasn't Dr. C. wise in predicting it?*

That might not be how this doctor would explain it, but it's how I understand it.

I truly believe that if a doctor thinks you can get well (or makes you believe that you can get well)—as both Dr. Roboz and Jon always have, as Peter always has—you believe it a bit too. I believe it a bit because my friends believe it—Jessie, Deena. The believing. There is something to it. If not in the long run, at the very least in finding comfort in the present. But sometimes in the long run too.

Dr. C. replaces hope with fear. Dr. C. should be stuck somewhere dealing with test tubes. Or at least given serious counseling. Keep this careless cruelty away from me. I'm a well of rage and I'm expelling this doctor after one false move.

What Dr. C. did to me is called "casting crepe," according to Jon. It's also known as "hanging crepe." *Crepe* (or *crape,* as it's sometimes spelled) is stiff shiny fabric that a woman was expected to wear for a year after losing her husband, back when society had rules about grieving. The medical expression *casting crepe,* as Google explains it, means "the doctor forecasts a bleak outcome to a patient." When he was an intern, Jon told me, he was taught that a doctor should never do it.

I can't avoid Dr. C. because this doctor is doing rounds. The next day, I bump into Dr. C. coming down the hall with a little troop of residents. The doctor is notably cheerful—maybe Dr. Roboz did some scolding. I did send a text complaining. I always have fantasies that busy Dr. Roboz is guarding my sanity. She has enough to do without doing that, but it wouldn't surprise me. Dr. C. examines me right there, listening to my heart in the hallway as if it's a fun thing to do.

I hate this doctor even more.

Peter and I move down to the oncology wing while CPX tanks my white cells. My niece Rachel comes from LA to visit and we spend the weekend doing a five-hundred-piece jigsaw puzzle of dog faces. I meet the friendly head of nurses from the transplant unit and she tells me that everyone loves working there. It's a special place. She offers, in a kind way, to shave my head when I'm admitted. She doesn't say *if* I'm admitted. I accept her offer. Eugene and Luc visit. Luc fits me for a wig. My head is small. "You have a ballerina head," says Luc.

On February 13, Peter gives me a valentine, a Victorian card of a couple in a small boat, the SS *Heart Throb,* Coney Island. The man's arm is tightly wrapped around the woman, their heads are snuggled together. The view is from their backs as they float into the Tunnel of Love. This is our metaphor. We will enter a dark tunnel but come out stronger and more in love. We tape it to the wall.

During my CPX treatment, Peter is busy e-mailing everyone, informing, updating, never indicating that anything but the most positive results are possible. How well I am doing, he says, how we're entering "the Tunnel of Healing." To his best friends Jim and Alice he writes, "We're signed on for this long and dangerous journey. As Delia is so completely healthy otherwise, we believe we will get that cure!" To his children, he composes a long note assuring them that I am an excellent candidate for a successful transplant. To Natasha, he writes, "I am very optimistic, and love and togetherness will help Delia pull through."

I don't see these notes. He's not a cheerleader with me. But he is calm, present, and never negative.

What amazes me, now that I review his e-mails, is that he never secretly wrote, *Oh God, this is a nightmare,* which it was.

The encounters with Dr. C. continue.

One morning, I ask Dr. C., "Do you by any chance know if Dr. Roboz is in the hospital today?"

"I have better things to do than keep track of the whereabouts of Dr. Roboz." The doctors in training and the PA are clustered around listening to this. Yes, this is how you talk to patients.

Another doctor introduces me to an intern and asks if the intern can track me for a few days. I say fine. The intern is around and about, here and there, chatting about this and that, and when he comes in to say goodbye, he says, "I bet you make it. You have good support. It makes a difference."

He's an intern, he knows almost nothing, but he does know something. His words reassure me. I feel my heart flutter. Maybe he's right.

I don't want to know my daily counts—whites, reds, platelets. I don't understand what the numbers mean and I can't turn myself into a person who tracks things, especially something that will only cause me more anxiety. A nurse wakes me at 6:30 or so every morning to take blood, and by the time the doctor does rounds, he or she has the results and can order a transfusion of reds or platelets if necessary.

Peter wants to track my counts. We arrange with doctors to write them on a piece of paper or tell them to him privately in the hall.

One morning when Dr. C. does rounds, Peter asks for my counts. Dr. C. says, "You don't need to know them, we're keeping track."

Trust the hospital to keep track? No. Never be in the hospital alone, if possible, even if you're getting fantastic care. Always have a double-checker present. Also, Dr. C. knows Peter is a doctor. Everyone knows because every time I introduce him, I add, "He's a doctor." I say it because if they know that, I feel more protected. Then they say politely, "Oh, what kind of doctor?" He says, "Psychiatrist," and that's sort of the end of it. He's just a psychiatrist. He merely deals with the mind. Still, I persist. I believe it will give me an edge. It's a fantasy, but it makes me feel better.

Dr. C. leaves the room, and Peter runs out and waylays the doctor, he told me later, near the nurses' station. Everyone can hear him say, "I'm Delia's husband and she has asked you to give me her blood counts. We have a right to know. And you have no right to treat us this way. You have no right to treat us disrespectfully."

It sounds very exciting. If I hadn't already been in love with him, I would have fallen in love right then.

Not looking at him, not apologizing, walking into the next patient's room, the doctor says, "We'll get you the numbers."

The PA shows up later and gives Peter a piece of paper with the counts.

I see Dr. C. only one more time.

At the end of my course of CPX, after the bone marrow biopsy and days waiting to hear results, sleeping only because they give me an antianxiety med, I'm sitting with Peter at the table in my room doing the last of the dog puzzle, and Dr. C. walks in. The doctor stands quite a distance away and says, without joy, "The CPX was successful. Your marrow is clean. There is no residual leukemia."

I still hate the doctor, but I'm happy. I'm going to Transplant.

*W*e are anxious to start. Excited, even. Feeling like good things can happen. Waiting for an available room, which doesn't turn up until eight that night.

10 WEST

BLOOD STEM CELL

&

BONE MARROW

TRANSPLANT UNIT

I arrive through the double doors by wheelchair, as patients do, pushed by an orderly. Peter is by my side with my roller bag. The door has many signs. NO LIVE FLOWERS OR PLANTS ARE PERMITTED ON THE UNIT. Two people with a line through them: PLEASE DO NOT ENTER UNLESS YOU ARE A VISITOR OF A PATIENT ON THIS UNIT. And a third: ANY VISITOR WHO HAS A FEVER, COLD, OR ANY KIND OF ILLNESS OR HAS BEEN EXPOSED TO ANY KIND OF CONTAGIOUS ILLNESS SHOULD NOT COME INTO THIS UNIT.

I am in the major leagues now. Everything up to this point, I will discover within days, was minor. A trifle. My CPX? A mere inconvenience. Now I find out what really being sick is, what trying to be cured truly involves.

Ten West is a plain U-shaped wing, its plaster walls painted beige, with a view at the end downriver of the 59th Street Bridge. The nurses' station at the center, bisecting the U, has access to both sides. The hall is notably quiet, not simply at eight p.m. but always. The rooms are filled, but there are rarely patients wandering about (mainly, I assume, because they are very weak). One other reason it's quiet—every room has an anteroom with an air lock. An air lock is meant to reduce any airborne infections. It prevents hall air getting into the patient's room. It also buffers sounds.

Only one couple walks the corridor, a man and woman. She is in a robe. A nurse sits at a computer along the corridor, entering notes. We cross at the nurses' station to my room on the left side. It's very small.

The welcoming nurse recites the rules for me and Peter in a rather rigid way. She informs Peter that he cannot use my bathroom. It is exclusively for the patient. He has to leave Ten West and find a public bathroom somewhere else. If he wants to spend the night, he can recline in the chair. "Can we get a larger room tomorrow, one with enough space for a daybed?" he asks.

She can't promise it. She will try. "We hope we can find something better for you."

We unpack my stuff. Peter tapes our Tunnel of Love valentine on the wall, stays awhile, kisses me, and reluctantly goes home for the night.

The next day, I do get a bigger room. It already has a daybed in it. We are enormously relieved.

The nice nurse shaves my head the next morning because the

chemotherapy will make my hair fall out anyway. I am now a bald woman in bed. The view out the window is of a concrete hospital roof. There is a round table, a TV, and a whiteboard that the nurses write on. Day 1, then 2, up and up. My counts are supposed to go on it too, but I ask them not to record them there, to tell Peter instead. The nurses write their own names and the names of the nurse's aide and the physician's assistant, all of which change with every shift. Diagonally from the bed, in a corner, is a reclining chair where visitors sit, because it is farthest from me. The nurses suggest I should sit there too as much as possible. Sitting up is better than lying down, and very quickly all I want to do is lie down.

I begin five days of "conditioning," a euphemism for, as Peter describes it, "high toxicity and torture." Each chemotherapy I had over the five days was toxic on its own, but the last, melphalan, is the one that leaves its mark.

Melphalan is supposed to make sure any remaining leukemia cells that might be hiding somewhere in my body are eradicated. I receive it through an IV drip. During this process, melphalan can destroy the inside of my mouth and throat. I misunderstand and believe it can destroy my entire digestive tract, but my mouth and throat are frightening enough. The only thing that counteracts its destructiveness and ensures its effectiveness, the nurse explains, is keeping my mouth freezing throughout the process. I have to ice my mouth for an hour before, and I have to chew ice during the entire infusion. Then I have to chew ice for an hour afterward. I am terrified the entire time. It's horrendous.

Once I survive melphalan, I am reliving it. The memory haunts my days in the hospital as I get weaker and weaker. I dream the fear at night. I can still taste the ice. Melphalan has brutal side effects. I can't keep anything down. I am constantly grabbing a plastic bowl to vomit in. I lose interest in food immediately. I can't taste it. I simply can't eat. I am too weak to get to the bathroom. This all happens quickly.

In the afternoons Peter leaves me with Linda, goes down to our apartment, showers, checks the mail, has some patient phone or video hours, and brings me back sorbet from the gelato place on the corner. After melphalan, I only like the purple flavors, like grape and blackberry. I don't actually like them, but I can tolerate a few bites. In the morning, breakfast arrives. I always try the cantaloupe, which is hard and out of season.

The pills. There are so many. Their names, with lots of syllables, are unpronounceable. They come in all sizes, some enormous and navy blue, some tiny and pink. Some I take once a day, some twice, some three times. Some are not pills but fluids injected into my mouth. It's relentless. They just keep coming. I count them later in my records: around thirty standing-order meds taken orally every day. The amounts fluctuate. Once I get the transplant, they'll have to give me other stuff to ward off graft-versus-host disease. Also, because my white count is now zero, they have to watch me closely and give me antibiotics at the slightest sign of a fever.

The pills start early, at 5:00 or 6:00 a.m., then more at 9:00, noon, 3:00, 6:00, and 9:00 p.m. I dread them. I have never had an easy time with pills, but with this nausea, I can't swallow them. I throw them up. I have to take them again. They are daily punctuation and failure. A constant drama. Sometimes I take them with water, sometimes I try yogurt or sorbet, sometimes applesauce. A pill. How bad can it be? It's like being visited again and again by demons.

There are infusions too. And transfusions. A bag of something going into my veins is often hanging from a pole next to my bed.

One day after melphalan, on February 26, when its side effects are just kicking in, I get my first donor transplant. "They hang this little bitty plastic bag on the IV, a yellowish plasma-like substance," as Peter describes it. These are my adult donor's actual stem cells. "It's exciting. Almost festive," he says.

"The feeling is you have done everything you can to get this working. I was happy," he insisted later. "Not one thing had gone wrong, although I felt terrible about how torturous it was for you. We were very optimistic."

The transfusion takes less than an hour. Dr. van Besien shows up. Dr. Roboz puts in an appearance. It's celebratory. Everyone is proud of how well I'm doing.

Peter to all my beloved girlfriends:

> Just want you to know that Delia's doing great—the donor marrow cells went in today just fine. She'll still be "slammed" as she puts it for a few more days, mostly sleeping it off, but that's the effect of last week's chemo build-up which should be diminishing over the next few days. No fevers, no reaction from the donor cells. Baby stem cells go in tomorrow. Hopefully she'll regain her energy to communicate in the next day or two. But she (and we) feel all the love coming from you!
> Love, Peter

From Julia to me, February 26:

> Dearest Delia,
> Peter sent on the extremely reassuring news about the result of your treatment yesterday. I was thinking of you so

much, on Sunday night, how nervous you might feel, and how much I wished I could be with you. And then, at 12:30 on Sunday night, Poppy went into labour (two weeks earlier than expected) and I drove up to London in the middle of the night. So, such a strange day yesterday, of love and hope flying across the Atlantic and toward St. Mary's Hospital in London, aware of two of the most loved and important women in my life going through huge challenges. How strange life is, and how relieved I feel this morning to get Peter's email. Take care of yourself, my darling, and I'll phone in a few days, when you've had time to recover a little more. Lots and lots of love, Julia xxxxx

Julia's daughter, Poppy, is having a baby at the same time that I am getting baby stem cells. She's giving birth and I am being reborn. Big things for both of us. But really, miracles or suffering, or miracles that involve suffering, they are all specific. I am cut off now. Being a patient in a hospital is being the center of the world—a very small world, but I am the definite center. Everyone is there for me. At the same time, I'm powerless. The center of the world but powerless.

The next day I get the second transplant, the umbilical cord blood stem cells. It goes in smoothly too.

With the impact of melphalan, and in spite of this good news, I stop eating. I am put on an intravenous diet and quickly sink into weakness, constant nausea, pill-dread, and despair.

This exchange between Meredith and Peter only two days after the transplant:

From Meredith to Peter, March 1:

Hi Peter,

I think of you both every waking hour. I hope you have support and are holding up through this really terrible period. I know from Delia's very brief emails that she is in bad shape. I know she is feeling horribly sick, and I can't imagine how horrible, or how hard it is for you to witness. I just pray the doctors feel the transplant went well and there haven't been setbacks. And that she is on track. It may be too early to know what's going on but I'd be grateful for a brief report when you're up to sending one.

Love,

Meredith

Peter to Meredith:

Hi Meredith—

Was just starting to write you back when, as if in answer, Delia suddenly stirred from sleep and said, "I definitely feel a little better."

Thankfully, all continues well medically. Delia had a brief episode of atrial fib yesterday, just as she experienced almost a year ago on the very first round of CPX-351. But none of the dreaded fevers, and no evidence of any rejection of those precious donor stem cells. The medical team says that this is just what a successful transplant looks like, that everything is on course. But yes, she's been miserable with nausea, not eating, fatigue, feeling depersonalized. That's pretty much from all the super-intense final week of chemo before the donor cells infusion. She's sleeping much of it off.

So let's hope that tonight's "better" suggests the misery will be abating in the next few days.

Through it all, we do take little walks in the halls, and watch *Seinfeld* episodes (each and every one is on Hulu), or take a look at other comedies.

I'm doing OK—yes, I hate her misery, as you do, and the helplessness of it. Yet I can stand outside it and remind Delia 100 times a day that everything, even the misery, is part of the healing path. We continue through the mysterious and scary Tunnel of Love.

Hopefully in a few days she'll have the wherewithal to talk to you on the phone, which I know will be a great comfort to her.

And soon we will all meet, on one coast or the other.

Love,

Peter

Peter keeps everyone posted. Alice and Gail M. write that they are doing tonglen, a Tibetan Buddhist meditation practice where one can take in suffering from another, transform it, and send out healing. Every day they both do it. It's comforting to think that my friends outside our little hospital entrapment are trying to help me heal.

Ten days after the transplant, the doctor doing rounds tells me my marrow is producing white cells. The transplant has taken root. The doctors call this "engrafting." I am sitting up in bed. I shoot my fist into the air. "Yes!" I shout.

I don't think I have ever yelled "Yes!" in my life, but there it is.

$\mathcal{P}$eter is writing the good news to everyone. Sometimes individually, sometimes in groups. "It is now ten days post–donor cell infusion, and just today there is solid evidence that the donor marrow is beginning to put some white cells into circulation. This is great news!"

His positivity, his refusal to let us feel or be beaten, is heroic. *Husband at bedside* is a note made every day by the attending doctor.

My "feeling better" is a blip. In spite of the transplant taking hold in my marrow, everything is not "going well." I remember this time in the hospital only in patches. Nurses coming in and out, the whiteboard—one name crossed off, another added on—doctors, transfusions, pills. Horrible memories of melphalan. Peter trying to coax me to eat. Peter reminding me to drink. Water, water, water. He is always pushing a water bottle my way. Even drinking water is difficult. Watching Ellen DeGeneres with Linda. Being held up by Linda to get to the bathroom.

Meredith arrives, unexpectedly and thankfully, from San Francisco. She explained later: "I just wanted to be there in case I was needed for anything. It was cold, it was winter, it was flu season. What if Peter got sick? I had to be there. What if something happened to him?"

Meredith recalled my state. "You weren't interested in anything in the outside world. No room in your brain for it. You perked up when I mentioned that I might take a long-term rental in New York. Once you noticed my very colorful scarf. 'Oh, I love that scarf,' you said. It was your voice. It was your real voice. I understood you were there. You would come to life every so often in small flashes like that. Mostly you were very quiet and very still. Linda and Peter were like small points of light in a dark universe. We were all waiting for you to rejoin the solar system."

One day, according to Meredith, I say, "I don't know what's going on. I don't even know what my immune system does."

"Don't bother to learn now, because you're getting a new one," Meredith says.

She said later, "Some days, you were detached in a way that was pretty remarkable. One day you had a big drip going into your arm. 'Oh, look at that,' you said. 'Isn't it amazing, they can just hang that stuff up and put it right inside of you.' You said it with such wonder, like it was someone else's arm and body you were talking about. At one point, you said, 'Am I bananas to be doing this?' as if you were asking about going on an extravagant vacation. I think you benefited from not knowing that much. If I asked something, you would say, 'I don't know, ask Peter. He's the man in charge.' Or sometimes it would be 'He's the one with the answers.'"

I do remember Meredith's scarf. And her flirtation with a semipermanent New York home. I remember she brought me a cupcake from Amy's Bread and I couldn't bring myself to eat it, which would have been unheard of in my healthy days. I remember her arrivals, a kind of life force blowing in.

Meredith: "Peter was so upbeat in the room. If he was concerned, he would say it only outside, in the little anteroom. And even then he would say it with a little gesture of his hand, a little waggle, as if to say, *It's just a minor thing*. Even when I knew it wasn't a minor thing.

"I would encourage him to take a break when I came. He did at least start taking a walk. He never wanted to leave. He would go home and shower. He was so sweet and encouraging. He treated the doctors so well—not a competitive thing. Never that kind of shit I see so often. He would always try to involve you. 'Isn't that right, Delia, did you hear what I'm telling Meredith? Look at the counts Delia has. Look how great she's doing.' He absolutely believed. I never introduced any doubt into the equation even when I felt it. To do so would have been an absolute violation of the emotional space Peter had unswervingly planted himself in."

Peter to Jon on March 3 (perhaps because they are both doctors, he is more frank than usual):

Jon—

All is going according to top expectations—the docs are VERY happy with all the transplant parameters thus far, as of Day +4.

Trouble is, one of the expectations is persistent nausea, fatigue and loss of appetite, and this has made Delia quite miserable for the last few days. It's more likely the build-up from the week of conditioning meds than anything from the transplant itself. She understands that all this misery is expectable, yet feels trapped in the hell of it until the nausea remits. Oh, and she had a brief return of A-fib for a few hours yesterday, just as she had last April. The heart rate has normalized, but that was scary as hell for a few hours. Yet we are keeping chins up, walking down the hall now and then, and reminding ourselves of the bright future this will bring. She's just started TPN [intravenous nutrition] tonight after eating virtually nothing for four days.

Hopefully she will be up to communicating at some point over the weekend.

I'm doing fine—I'm on the journey, too, but it's not going through my body and marrow. Just my soul.

Will give her your love until you can do it directly, and our love back to you and Kate.

Love, Peter

Random musings PS (forgive my first draft late at night-itis): Because it's not a heart transplant, which thanks to that famous, visible organ makes it unmistakable to both patient and all concerned what the existential experience must be of being snatched from the brink of death through the miracle of organ donation, I think Bone Marrow/Stem Cell Transplant does not so obviously have the same existential reputation, so a certain relative nonchalance is expected of patient and loved ones. But the existential shock is equivalent, and the body and (as we Jungians are prone to say) the Unconscious (that is, the soul) Knows. And it is screaming, as Delia is inwardly doing right now.

*E*very day a tall male doctor comes into the room, stands on the side of the bed near my head, and says, "What did you eat today?"

"Nothing," I say. Or "A little gelato."

He is managing my nutrition and, having established that the intravenous feeding should continue, he leaves. The encounter takes maybe fifteen seconds. One day, I say in despair, "This is rough." And he, staring down at me intently, says, "This is war."

One day Meredith tells me, "You were in the ICU."

I don't know what she's talking about.

Apparently, on March 6, she explains, only nine days after the actual transplant, my A-fib got much worse. The doctors increased my metoprolol, the drug that controls this, to no avail, and I was moved to the ICU. I was there five days.

I have no memory of this lost time. Not an image. Not a sound. Not a speck. In my conscious mind, I have never seen an ICU.

"When you were in the ICU," Meredith tells me, "we all had to wear protective gear. There was a small room to go through before entering your room. That's where we had to sterilize our hands and put on plastic shields to cover our faces. That little room announced how deadly serious everything was. I was terrified that I'd bring some bug from the outside world into your room. I stayed off subways and put a small towel on the seat when I took an Uber to the hospital. I was always super-scared. What if I had something that you got? We couldn't get close to you, hold your hand."

Meredith and Linda regale me with tales of my behavior at the end of my ICU stay.

"They took you for an MRI and I went with you," says Meredith. "Abdomen and chest. That was when you got so upset. You didn't want to be in the machine. They couldn't complete the MRI. You told them, 'Fuck you.'"

Linda, who had not been at the MRI but had witnessed a certain amount of my behavior before in the ICU, adds, "You were saying that to everyone."

It is exciting to hear this, that I caused a ruckus. I'm not sure why. Surely partly from the safety of its being over. Partly being a patient is so confining. I was glad to hear I "acted up."

Then, right in the middle of my swearing at everyone, according to Linda, I stopped and said, "Did Binky get a new car?" Binky was a close friend of Nora's.

Linda and I start laughing. "I said, 'Did Binky get a new car?'"

Later—a long while later—Meredith told me the whole story of the MRI, which she felt was too traumatizing to tell me then. Peter was at our apartment having a shower, then doing a Zoom with a patient, and the transport staff came early, so Meredith went with me from the ICU to the MRI suite. She was waiting outside for them to complete the scan and heard me yelling and screaming. "Stop this, stop this right now! Fuck you! Fuck you all!" Over and over I screamed. One of the techs came out and said, "Miss Ephron seems upset. We're halfway through the scan and she won't let us finish."

"They asked me to help calm you down," said Meredith. "You had kicked off the covers and torn off your hospital gown. You were lying there completely exposed, naked, kicking and flailing, wildly punching your arms into the air, saying, 'Stop, no more of this shit.' I kept trying to calm you, but it had little effect.

"As you were finally starting to calm down, Peter walked through the door. He practically dove for a blanket that was nearby and covered you with it, tucking it all around you, caressing your arms to soothe you. All he was interested in was preserving your dignity, covering and protecting you. Then he said calmly but very forcefully, 'There is no need to continue this. Let's just take her back to the room.'

"On the elevator going upstairs, now to the regular transplant wing, Ten West, he held on to the blanket, keeping you covered. The staff got you to a room and transferred you to a bed. And you fell asleep.

"I was shaking," said Meredith. "I started telling Peter how traumatic it had been but then thought maybe he didn't want to hear it. Peter said, 'She's delusional from all the steroids she's been on.'

"That made sense to me. All the time I had been imagining that you were saying exactly what you'd wanted to say for weeks to everyone throughout your whole time in the hospital. You'd finally let the interior voice out. I was comforted by the fact that you were 'delusional.' That wasn't you at all.

"That incident is seared in my memory, especially the image of Peter diving for the blanket to cover you up."

It's peculiar to hear this, to try to comprehend my level of distress. It feels as if it's a story about another person. And I'm sad to hear about what I put Meredith and Peter through.

About being naked: There was some point in this, fairly early on, where I lost all sense of modesty or privacy. Not eating, getting weaker, having a constant parade of nurses taking my vitals, feeding me transfusions and pills, losing all sense of taste and constantly throwing up, I had no sense of my own physicality. I was a victim of my body's going crazy.

On my return from the ICU, with my A-fib successfully treated, I am given a small room and a minder. A nurse's aide sits with me all day to make sure I don't climb out of my bed. The rails are all up; still, I am trying to get out. I don't remember this either. Peter can't sleep in the room, not enough space. He talks it over with the head nurse. A larger room like the one we had been in before I went to the ICU, he insists, is better for me, one with a bigger window, more light, cheerier, and with a daybed so he can stay. Plus, he tells the head nurse, he could help the minder. Finally, she agrees. He considers that one of his biggest triumphs, getting us back into a bigger room. Although I think his biggest triumph is his constancy, his refusal to believe I would die or to let me die later, when I was begging him to let me go.

He does not let anyone know about this early ICU stay when my heart is acting up or this MRI traumatic incident. He is tracking my numbers in my blood count to see if the stem cell transplant is working. He believes the numbers because the medical team keeps saying, "As long as the bone marrow graft is working, she'll get better." And the numbers show that the transplant is working. Everyone assures Peter—Dr. van Besien, his associates, and the nurses who did nothing else but transplants on Ten West.

Right in the middle of my A-fib, March 7, he writes Heather:

> Hi Heather—
> There is good news in that the donor marrow is beginning to put just a few white cells into the circulation. Nausea and general discomfort are easing, but it's still a tough road, as she's not eating yet and is getting all nutrition IV. Yet her spirits are good. We're told that if the white count continues its slow rise, EVERYTHING gets better fast!
> Will send your love to Delia and keep you posted.—Peter

From Heather to Peter, March 8:

Peter, That is such such wonderful news. I hate to think of Delia in the state you describe, hearing about her being so vulnerable makes me want to come and stand guard outside the hospital. But I will focus on the long term, when she's well again and back with us. The world feels off balance knowing she's not in her apartment on Tenth Street. Please give my love. And do let us know if there's anything we can do for you as well; I know being the primary support for someone going through what Delia is going through is difficult and tiring. We're so grateful to you for all you give her. Love, Heather

From Deena to Peter, March 8:

If Delia is well enough to read this—please tell her I miss her terribly right now because I have an issue with my book agent and don't know exactly what to do and so would have, in the past, called Delia and she would have told me and I would have done exactly what she said. We tend to tell each other what to do—both of us not really taking that kind of directive from anyone but the other. It will have to wait until I see her but it will take a nice long chat when she is feeling more herself.

I hold only good thoughts for both of you and lots of love, Deena

$\mathcal{M}$eredith flies back to San Francisco, thinking I'm over the hump. But mentally, I'm deteriorating.

As days go by, I remember this: I would watch the clock, just watch minutes tick by.

A random assortment of notes in the records in the days following the ICU: *Patient can't identify her palm. Patient can't spell* world *backwards. This patient is at high risk for morbidity and mortality given the underlying malignancy, comorbidities, and current treatment. Continue to monitor carefully for chemotherapy and post-transplant toxicity.*

That repeats again and again. *Occasional difficulty speaking and using her Chapstick. Patient very anxious on visit preferring writer to speak with husband. Patient has altered mental status today; tried to climb out of bed last night; today can't answer questions such as are you short of breath, are you hungry; simply looks away and says nothing; cannot carry on any conversation.*

Then on March 13: *The nurses found her incontinent of urine and saying she wanted to die.* March 14: *Patient says she wants this to end multiple times but not answering questions.*

Up to that time, there were occasional notes: *Patient says she's going to die.* This is the first time I notice them reporting me saying, "I want to die."

I wonder if they quoted me properly. I thought this came later.

I am, according to Dr. van Besien, suffering from toxic-metabolic syndrome, which basically means my brain is affected because my body is not eliminating toxic byproducts, whatever they are. It can cause anything from nothing to death.

On March 26, 2018, at 1:27 p.m., Peter wrote to friends and family:

Dear Ones—

After 49 days at Weill Cornell and all signs that the engrafted bone marrow is putting out healthy blood cells, Delia is being discharged from the hospital tomorrow! Before going home, the transplant program puts people up at the Helmsley Medical Tower Hotel across the street, for 2 weeks of day hospital at the out-patient clinic, 9 am to 5 pm. We are deliriously happy that the MDs say "it worked." Yet Delia is still miserable most of the time with fatigue and nausea, starting to eat but still very little, and will still be on IV nutrition for a while. We are reassured that this is just what recuperation is supposed to look like. Visits and communication are still very limited, so email Delia with copies to me and I will read everything to her. In the weeks and months ahead we will celebrate without restraint, and together with all!

Love from Peter and Delia

From Jessie:

> Thank you dearest dearest Peter.
> A miracle. xo

From Deena:

> What great news to wake up to! And on opening day for all 30 teams. An abundance of riches. Grateful and happy.
> xxxooo
> Deena

From Peter's close friend Alice, March 26:

> Peter. Thank you for the update and glad for the good news about Delia's recovery.
> Please tell her that when she is up for it, I intend to pull up the rug in the living room, put on some good Motown and DANCE away the night.
> She reminds me to live fully.
> Much love to you both. Alice

From Natasha:

> Wow, wow, wow.
> AMAZING news.
> Go Delia GO!!!
> Can't wait to visit in April.
> Much love.
> Natasha

From Julia, March 29:

> Dear Delia and Peter,
> This is the most wonderful news, bless your cotton socks, Delia.
> I got my ESTA visa today, which made me very excited at the thought of being with you this time next week. I really can't wait.
> The sun was setting tonight, and dusk descending as I crossed Bigsweir bridge, and all along the riverbank I saw dots of light from the hurricane lamps of the men who come to fish for Elvers (the eels, very popular in Japan). I was en route to Tori's house, the amazing baker you met and mother of now six who lives right at the top of an almost perpendicular hill called the Freedom. I was delivering a wicker cot for one of the twins that she'd given birth to that week. When I arrived it was like a scene from *Little Women,* her other children (all under 13) so excited, chopping vegetables and laying the table for supper.
> So, am packing tonight, as Poppy and Sam here for Easter and I don't want to get over-excited. I will await your orders as to whether to get my taxi to E 10th or the hospital suite.
> Much love to you both.
> J xxxx

The stories of life in Wales sound more and more like fairy tales, a place of magic and no place I will ever see again. In spite of my discharge to Helmsley, a marker of recovery, I am withdrawing almost completely from the world.

Linda and Peter pack me up. Peter takes the Tunnel of Love

valentine off the wall. It has protected us. I sit in the bed watching them. I am too weak to help, too weak to walk. I don't remember being happy, although I must have been. February 5 to March 26. Almost fifty days in the hospital. My cell phone feels too heavy to hold. I am not myself in any way, not able to do almost anything alone. Transport arrives. I am assisted into a wheelchair and pushed through an underground passage to Helmsley. I am still cowering at the enormous consumption of pills. My dread of them is growing. I still have melphalan memories every day. I am still not eating. Peter is given elaborate instructions of how to administer intravenous food supplements. It's a Rube Goldberg–ian task to connect all the parts to each other and to me. It feeds me at night while I sleep.

The Helmsley is a pleasant place whose existence is to serve Weill Cornell patients. It's sort of old-fashioned in style, and comforting, with drapes and comfy upholstered furniture. Every day, transport arrives and takes me via underground to the day clinic, where they take my blood and sometimes give me transfusions. My arms are speckled with red because I still have a low platelet count.

Jill visits. She is my friend-daughter who is also my friend-mother because I aspire to her bravery and travel fearlessness. She does not think I look terrible. In fact, she is blown away by my skin. "Your skin is so beautiful," she says. "Plump and dewy. Smooth, almost glowing. Your skin looks like skin women pay millions of dollars to get."

This is mysterious. It is the beginning of many compliments I get on the skin of my disappearing body. I have now lost about twenty pounds, and if I wore clothes, as opposed to pajamas, I would definitely be down two sizes. Apparently the cord blood stem cells can, for want of a better word, seep into your skin and give you the soft clear skin of a baby. Sort of. Well, enough that people start to mention how my face has no lines.

"You were in misery," she says. "And tired. I only stayed a short time." I tell her about the pills, that I can't stand them, that there are hundreds, that they are torturing me.

I have a fantasy that I could be hypnotized out of this misery. That a hypnotist could hang a pocket watch on a chain in front of my eyes, swing it back and forth, and say, "When I count backward from ten, you will love pills. You will never vomit pills. You will never have trouble swallowing a pill. They will taste as delicious as maple walnut creams, your favorite chocolate."

Jill can turn up anything in a second. She offers to find me a hypnotherapist. Maybe someone can put me in a trance to take pills. The woman she finds isn't a watch-swinging type. Is there even such a thing? Jill finds more a meditator, and I want a quick fix. Hypnotize me to swallow pills, please. We give up on that idea.

My text to Dr. Roboz on March 30:

It is a particular kind of hell to come back from this. Weakness and fear and trauma.

Dr. R. texts back:

You will bounce back strong and fit and fabulous and then write the best screenplay ever and Julia Roberts will play me. 😇

Looking at my records, I understand now why she was optimistic. My most recent bone marrow showed successful engrafting.

My counts, while still way under normal, were climbing. But my body was in revolt.

At the end of March, I am released to leave Helmsley to go home. I don't recall the marvel of this or the car ride downtown or any joy in seeing my beloved Tenth Street whose trees were in spring bloom and which had always brought me comfort.

Julia arrives—Julia, who never fails to raise my spirits—but truly I am feeling connected to no one.

I am sliding into a deep depression.

I have never before been clinically depressed. Anxious and worried, yes. Frightened, yes. Dislocated, yes. Sad, yes. But I have never ever felt deep in my bones a despair, an isolation from everyone, a wish to be dead. I feel all that now.

E-mail from Julia to Deena after Julia arrives in New York City, April 4:

Hi Deena,

So, update for you: in many ways, it is such a relief to see her, though daunting too in ways I will try to describe. It feels like foreign territory, which I suppose all health crises are. Although she has lost all that lovely hair, in some ways I had prepared myself for her looking much thinner and more frail. (She is still fed, mainly on intravenous food, but Peter is trying to coax her back to ordinary food, the most successful so far is Jell-O, and peaches.)

Please understand here, I am trying to agree with Peter that the good news, and it IS good news, is that the actual bone marrow transplant has taken, but the shock for me is how depleted she seems. Very, very tired. We have, for instance, only exchanged about two sentences today, and she seems a little distraught at how weak and out of it she feels. I've told her absolutely no need to make any effort for me—I've actually brought part of my book to edit, but I think she is upset she can't be more her old self.

She told me yesterday she would never have gone through this procedure had she realized how awful it would be. Having said that, she recognizes it is early days, and it will take a good six months to feel normal again.

I feel I (and you when you come) can be useful here, shopping and an extra pair of hands for Peter, who has been so magnificent, and who is determinedly optimistic, but who must be under enormous strain.

I'm sure it will be a wonderful boost to her spirits to see you. Hope this is helpful.

love Julia x

Julia goes out a bit every day to walk around the city and do some final research for her novel. She always brings me a present— a pendant, a scarf, something. But all I remember is one moment on her last day. I'm flopped diagonally across my bed and say to her, "I'm done. It's over."

Julia leaves thinking she will never see me again.

Peter asks Gail M. to stay with me when he goes out briefly, giving her strict instructions to make me sit up periodically, not to let me lie down all the time. She told me later, "I have never seen anyone sicker." She makes me sit up once but then gives in to my continual refusal to do it again.

On April 16, we go in for an appointment at the transplant clinic. On this day, VB is away and we see Dr. Peter Abdelmessieh.

He is a fellow for a year with VB, and I like him. His long hair is pulled back in a ponytail; he has a trim beard, warm dark eyes, and a wonderfully friendly smile. He's youngish; late thirties, early forties. We know a bit about him, that he's engaged to be married. It comes out in conversation, but he doesn't talk about himself. He knows I'm the patient.

I'm sitting there when he walks in—it's clinic room 26, where I first met VB. Seeing how distressed I am, picking it up from my face, he says, "What is it you want to do right now?" This is not a conventional opening doctor question.

I point to the exam table. "I want to lie down."

"Okay, sure."

I curl up on my side on the table and look up at him looking down at me. I'm relieved to be horizontal. Dr. Abdelmessieh says, "I hope you don't mind, but you're not leaving the hospital today."

Dr. Mayer, one of the attending physicians on VB's team, comes in and concurs that I should be rehospitalized. He leaves and returns a few minutes later. "There's a room for her."

I know I am coming back to die.

A note in my hospital records on readmission: *Failure to thrive*. Peter says that means, in hospital-speak, that I'm starving to death.

April 17, 2018

Hi Peter,

Are things moving in the right direction? I've emailed Delia but haven't heard back so don't want to bother her again. Just feeling a little uneasy that I haven't had a report in a while. Hope my inquiries aren't annoying.

Much love

Meredith

Peter spins things positively.

Hi Meredith—

Things were improving very gradually last week in terms of swallowing pills and bites of food, but then over the weekend Delia started spitting things up again. So yesterday at the outpatient clinic they decided that she needs a full workup of the digestive problems, and that this would best be done as an in-patient, so she was readmitted to 10 West last evening, which we are both very relieved about. They are hydrating her and getting her ready for an endoscopic upper GI biopsy and lower GI studies to see what is going on.

She perked up a bit today from the hydration, and they can give her most meds IV, but she is still throwing up. She is still sleeping much of the time but is completely present when she wakes up, although she can't sustain conversation for long due to fatigue and as you noticed is not checking her email, voice mail or texts. So she is still on TPN nutrition. I think when they get to the bottom of what is disrupting the GI system and treat it, her energy will pick up.

The maddening paradox is that this is all on the heels of a perfect report on the genomics of her bone marrow biopsy, showing NO remaining chromosomal abnormalities that had been driving her leukemia.

Don't ever think you are annoying to either of us! Your presence and love are palpably making a difference.

Will keep you posted.

Love,

Peter

E-mail, me to Jessie, April 17:

Back in the hospital. Feeling awful.

Jessie to Peter and me:

> Would you like Bryan and me to visit you in the hospital?
> We are here.
> If not, Peter, fill me in and what this chapter is.

This chapter is my last. I haven't gotten any better at eating. I'm still nauseous and vomiting. In addition to these being chemotherapy effects, as Peter told Meredith, they are also symptoms of graft-versus-host disease, the donor cells attacking my gastrointestinal tract. My body is fighting the transplant. Or, rather, the transplant is fighting my body.

To confirm it, they give me a gastroscopy, which involves five to ten minutes of sedation and a tube down my esophagus. They do a biopsy of my stomach lining.

I am too debilitated to understand what is happening.

I call Jon and ask him to come to the hospital, and he does. I am lying limply in bed. This is all I can do. There is a commode next to the bed. I cannot walk to the bathroom. Jon is friendly with Dr. Roboz. From the beginning, with my permission, they have regularly discussed my case. "Ask her to put me on something like a morphine drip," I tell him. I am actually allergic to morphine, so I figured that would just make me sicker and not necessarily kill me or kill me but torture me at the same time. So "something *like* morphine."

Jon sits down on the edge of the bed. "You're not sick enough," he says. Apparently, a doctor can't kill someone because he, she, or they ask him to. If you are on the way out, a doctor can give you something to ease your suffering, which might also ease you out. But I must be on the way out. If *I'm* not sick enough,

I can't imagine who is. He talks to me about depression. He says my depression will break and that might happen just after it gets darkest.

Jon and Peter privately confer about my state. "We had the same view," said Peter, "that you were not of sound enough mind to make that decision. Your mind was clouded by having low oxygen, you couldn't think clearly, and you were completely traumatized." Peter added, "You didn't have your adult mind available. You can't let a child make that decision."

I am on antidepressants—they are some of my thousands of pills a day—but they don't make a whit of difference.

Again and again I ask Peter to take me out. I'm on the bed, and he's in the chair. I plead weakly. "Please. Please."

He says, "Everything is going to be okay."

I also tell Linda I want to die, which upsets her. Actually, I upset everyone.

I can sit up if someone cranks up the back of the bed. I sit there with my eyes closed, looking at blackness, thinking this is death. This is what it is.

The doctors bombard me with steroids to attack this graft-versus-host disease. An infusion plus pills. More pills.

On April 23, seven days after readmission, I wake up and can barely breathe. My oxygen is low. All the fluid they are giving me through my veins to feed me is filling my lungs. This is called fluid overload. The graft-versus-host disease is getting better, but my treatment could be killing me.

I am put on oxygen. I do not have pneumonia, but I might get pneumonia. I believe I have pneumonia, though. Pneumonia, old man's friend, yes, please. They immediately put me in a tent to get my oxygen saturation up. After that, I have a large mask on my face. My oxygen blood levels (the amount of oxygen carried by blood)—known as PO_2—are being tracked every second.

Peter stays up night after night tracking my PO_2 on the screen and watching me breathe. If my oxygen level drops below 90, even with supplemental oxygen, that means the fluid is winning the battle. "It's like drowning," he later said.

Gail M. comes to see me. She sits next to the bed, right near my head. We whisper. I beg her to help me die. I beg her to convince Peter. "Please, Gail," I say again and again. "Talk to him, help me."

"It would destroy Peter," Gail M. tells me. "It would be awful."

"Oh, please," I say, "do you know how quickly someone would scoop him up? He's great."

"He's a hoverer," says Gail M. "Hoverers don't want to hover over a lot of people. Takes a lot of energy and worry, and you have to tolerate a lot of resistance."

"I don't know if I love him."

How horrible is this? How could I think this? But I do. He's a stranger across a room. He's in the way. I am cut off from any feeling except an intense misery and desire to die.

"I don't love him," I say.

"You can't know what you feel now."

"I can't imagine ever having that feeling again."

"That will change," says Gail M. She also talks about depression, as Jon did, how you could break out of it just when it seemed bleakest. I don't listen, really. I want out and no one is helping me.

Darling Peter. Guiding me, guarding me, staying up all night watching me breathe, reviewing every move the doctors make for going on sixty-plus days now, and I'm saying, "I don't know if I love him." That's depression. A complete disconnection.

I understand suicide now, how people leave behind families, lovers, friends, children. All I want is blackness. An empty screen.

Generally speaking, Gail M. said later, if Peter said anything positive, like I was getting better, I would jump on him, annoyed: "How do you know?" He would smile. "Well, we'll just have to see." He was very much *Okay, you can feel that way.* He was non-confrontational. I was a skinny, sick raging animal. I was feral.

Gail M. has a serious talk with Peter outside in the hall. She tells him again that she has never seen anyone as sick as me. He assures her that he wouldn't continue to put me through this if he didn't believe it was working. *This is what a successful transplant looks like.* When the doctors tell Peter that, he believes them. He is watching my numbers, my reds, my whites, my platelets. I am getting sicker, but my marrow is healthy, my numbers are climbing.

Some doctor will help me die. I ask Peter to see if Dr. Kurth, my internist, will visit.

E-mail, Peter to Dr. Kurth:

> Dear Becky,
> Delia is now on the Bone Marrow Transplant unit at Weill Cornell, day +60 with good engraftment, but dealing with several threatening complications. She is very scared just now and very much hopes you can come see her as soon as you can. I'm with her constantly.
> With much gratitude,
> Peter and for Delia

After her office hours, Dr. Kurth arrives. Dr. Rebecca Kurth, who is in her fifties, is a force—a clear, thoughtful, and exacting doctor. She has the kind of determination that makes me think she runs five miles a day. Actually, she seems like someone who could run the army. She once told me, "I can be abrupt sometimes. If that happens, let me know." I was pretty blown away by that bit of honesty. It endeared her to me forever. She has taken care of me for many years. She came to my apartment at 3:30 a.m. after Jerry died and sat with me for several hours in my bedroom waiting for his body to be taken away. Dr. Kurth was at Peter's and my wedding in the hospital when I was beginning my first chemo treatment.

I tell her I want to die, and she talks to me about "reinvention." Or "regeneration." I can't remember which or if it was another word entirely, and neither does she. "It must have been a word that came to mind when I was sitting next to you and inspiring you not to give up," said Dr. Kurth. "Words have so much power for you that I probably reached deep into my archives and pulled out something that would resonate with you. I knew you needed somebody you trusted to tell you that there was real hope and to not give up."

I am going to come back stronger, renewed, Dr. Kurth insists again and again. I called her to help me die, and I get nowhere with her. I get the opposite, regeneration not capitulation. She could not be more positive or kinder.

On April 26, ten days after my readmission, everything blows up. I am still on oxygen and the lung doctor advises a bronchoscopy to see if I have a fungal lung infection.

I refuse. I don't say it firmly, I say it wildly: *No, no, no. Please, no.*

A bronchoscopy involves being anesthetized and intubated, and it's possible that I would die from the procedure while intubated. I don't want to be intubated. I don't want this regardless of what it involves. No more treatment. I am done.

It's a mess of a day, full of friends. Jessie, worried, is visiting. Linda, distressed, is caring for me but feeling helpless. Natasha is here from California, having spent the day talking to editors who want to publish her book. A day of great excitement for her, but if she mentioned it, I don't remember. Death is the subject in the room. Peter consults with the lung doctor. She could not assure him that I would survive. I might not come out of the procedure alive, she says. He tells her we refuse.

"I wouldn't want you to die unconscious with a tube in you," Peter said later. "But I didn't decide anything ever without working with the team. I did make this decision with Dr. van Besien. He agreed. Great physicians know how to weigh the cost of doing all that science. VB didn't know if you had a fungal infection, but thought it was highly unlikely and we didn't need to risk killing you to find out."

I am frantic and sick and desperate to die. But see how muddled I am. I want to die but I don't want to die intubated. I'm saying no to something that could kill me while I beg for them to kill me.

While Peter is saddled with the responsibility of what course of action to take and sorting through all the possibilities, I am unaware of what he is experiencing. I don't even care anymore. I am done with tests.

A nurse walks in, stands at the foot of the bed, and says, "All the nurses agree with you about not having the bronchoscopy."

They agree with me? I am stunned. How extraordinary. I don't even answer. I simply stare. Does she mean that, since I'm dying, it's the right move, why bother with a test? Or does she mean it's simply unnecessary? Either way, they are on my side, and, how astonishing, the nurses weighed in.

Natasha about that day:

> When you were saying, "I just want to die," "I want this
> to be over," "I can't take this anymore," Jessie and Peter were
> very calm and boundaried with you. It was like you were a car
> careening off the tracks and every time you did, they would
> put up the guard rails to hold you in place. So in that way
> you were childlike. Almost like a tantrum. I remember being
> surprised that you were so blunt. I think I came and sat next
> to you on the bed—I was wearing a mask and a hair cap—
> and maybe I held your hand. Would they have let me get that
> close to you? Anyway, I was trying really hard not to cry or
> seem shaken by you and I remember you looking straight at
> me and telling me that you just wanted to die. You were in
> distress. You were sort of moving back and forth. Not a lot
> but kind of like a child having a bad dream where they thrash
> from side to side. You also told me you were getting tired and
> that I should go. You were incredibly matter-of-fact. No edit
> button—like a child.
>
> Peter was wearing his usual sort of outfit, dark pants and
> maybe a blue or black polo shirt and tennis shoes. He was
> steady, but he looked tired. His eyes were hollowed and I
> thought to myself "Who is taking care of Peter?" because he
> needs comfort and sustenance and support too. He never ever
> wavered (at least to me in our email exchanges, phone calls
> or that day in the hospital when we stood outside your door)
> in his certitude that you would make it. The setback was this
> gastric infection and he said once they figure out exactly what
> that was and how to effectively treat it you would be able to
> come back home and continue to recover. His words and his

way were very comforting. He was most definitely the light-house that we all needed, guiding your friends but especially you through that horrific experience.

On that day, April 26, in the morning, I had texted Dr. Roboz: Please let me go. I can't take another pill. Please.

Into this chaos—Natasha holding back tears; Linda, weepy, believing I am lost; Jessie and Peter trying to rein me in; me refusing further treatment and begging to die—into this chaos in late afternoon Dr. Roboz arrives, looking her usual glamorous in her white doctor coat, high heels, earrings, necklace, black hair to her shoulders, charmingly coiffed. "What's going on?" she says, as if she can't imagine what has gotten into me.

I spill it all. How awful I feel, that I won't do the bronchoscopy. I want out. I can't take another pill, I can't take another pill, I can't take another pill. I say that over and over. I want to die.

What I'm saying sounds strong, but I am nearly a skeleton, limp as a rag, on oxygen, unable to stand up without help, hardly able to sit up, my voice barely over a whisper. Dr. Roboz listens. "Give me forty-eight hours," she says, "and if I get somewhere, give me another forty-eight."

The next thing I recall is waking up. The room seems bright and friendly. I'm not hooked up to oxygen. Peter, looking tired and handsome, is sitting across the room. My depression is gone, almost magically, like someone waved a wand, and I know instantly I'm starting to heal.

Give me forty-eight hours, and if I get somewhere, give me another forty-eight. Hope and an endgame in one sentence. I often think about that. How close I came and how she honored my pain but still believed they could save me.

I have no idea what she and VB decided to treat me with. Later, Peter explained, it was maximum diuretics to flush all that fluid from my lungs. Peter sat up all night watching my oxygen levels, tracking my PO_2, willing it to stay up. "If it went down a little, I would turn up the oxygen, then tell the nurse what I'd done.

"It was close to forty-eight hours," said Peter, "when the nurse walked in and said, 'Let's try turning the oxygen down a bit.' She did, and you stayed saturated." He shook his head, wondering at it. "You stayed saturated. At ninety-five percent. That was the biggest sigh of relief. And nothing else was wrong with your lungs. That assessment was correct. It was a great moment."

The nurse tests me off and on for a while, but my lungs are fine, and whatever it is Dr. Roboz and Dr. van Besien came up with, it has emptied my lungs of fluid and cured my intestinal problem. I no longer need oxygen and am once again breathing, as the hospital puts it, "room air."

$\mathcal{P}$eter's daughter, Melina, has a baby girl somewhere in here—the world outside this room barely exists for me. I can't even pin down when this was. I know now it was April 25. Momentous things happening in other people's lives—it's as if they are taking place in another solar system.

But now I am stabilizing. The depression is gone, the terror too, and Deena is here from California.

I start eating again just as she arrives. I am handling pills a bit better. I am taking them with seltzer. "I remember the pills being constant," said Deena. "Nurses were always coming in. 'Now it's time to take two more.' You would say, 'Do I have to?' You looked horrendous," she added. "It wasn't just that you were bald. Your skin had a pallor, you were so thin."

It isn't easy for Deena to be here. Her grown daughter is disabled, and she has to arrange mountains of help to leave home, and I am so happy to see her. My spirits are rising. Peter, confident I am improving, leaves for San Francisco for a few days. He is excited to meet his new granddaughter but still reluctant to leave me.

"I wouldn't have gone if you weren't out of the woods. Not only were you breathing, you were eating. I left you in great hands with Deena." Peter quoted VB: "'When the bone marrow graft works, everything else gets better.'"

Everything is getting better.

Hard-boiled eggs. I don't know why I want them but I do.

Every morning, Deena comes to the hospital and brings me two hard-boiled eggs. I like them. I can taste them. I can keep them down. It's exciting to see these two eggs. Exciting to peel them. To actually eat them. After a short while, I ask VB how many hard-boiled eggs a day I am allowed to eat. He says, "Six." I believe he's probably fine with eight or ten. I'm sure he knows it's a short obsession. He seems a little surprised by the question.

Deena is a calm person. Actually, I think she would argue with me about that. But there is an order to her. She is always pulled together, thoughtful, and a deep thinker and writer about the things we both like to think about: why people behave the way they do. She is very calming to me.

For hours, Deena and I discuss a novel she is starting. I help her hash it out. My brain is working. We have always in the past noodled our projects together. It feels magical to concentrate, to get excited about characters, plot, to help spark her, to give back when I have been doing nothing these past months but let the love and care from everyone else pour into me.

"We would talk," said Deena. "Then you would say, 'I have to close my eyes.'"

We order dinner from an Italian restaurant in the neighborhood, and Deena picks up the delivery down in the hospital lobby. I eat a tiny bit of that too, some pasta pomodoro. Some fish. Not a lot, but some.

Deena and I have been friends for thirty-eight or so years. She was close to Jerry too. There is nothing I have done in life during that time that I haven't discussed with her. But now we are together in this hospital room eight to ten hours a day. Deena said, "What we experienced that week was just the essence of what a true friendship is. It was sort of as if you and I had gone on a trip together. It deepened our friendship in such a profound way." It was, I think, my vulnerability, her having to assist with prosaic tasks, and, mostly, simply the amount of time we were together. Conversations with purpose, conversations with depth, conversations that meandered. Silence. Sleep. Yes, even after years of endless phone calls and long lunches, we broke through to another level of comfort.

I can't get out of bed alone when she arrives. By the time she leaves, five days later, I can accomplish that, although Deena stands close by. She has to walk me to a toilet. The physical therapists, Joe and Jessica, have me standing and swaying. Standing and simply swaying is difficult. Jessica also puts Post-Its on the floor for me to step on, forward and back. My strength is minimal. I have no muscle tone, but I begin to use the rollator again, and, with Deena, I walk the seemingly long journey to the end of the hall. We look out the window at the tugboats, barges, and occasional tour boats on the East River. We appreciate the light on the water, the life on the bridge.

"The week gave me so much hope," said Deena. "Every day you got so much better."

Sometime during my last days in the hospital, either from Peter's reading my counts or some casual glance at the lab work, Peter and I realize that my blood is now type A.

Type A. It pops out at me.

I have always had type O blood. My marrow has always produced type O blood, but this new marrow is producing type A blood. This transplant has changed my blood type. What a shock. What an absolute astonishment. I have a different blood type.

It doesn't seem possible. And yet it is. O to A. That more than anything symbolizes the hugeness of what I am going through.

Text from me to Dr. Roboz, May 12, 2018, 9:32 a.m.:

Think it is all going well. Home!!!

part seven

Home

May 12, 2018

I am shy to enter my beloved building in such a frail state.

"Hi, Sam," I say brightly to the doorman as Peter pushes me in the wheelchair through the lobby to the elevator. Sam says, "Hi, Ms. Ephron." And that's it. I don't explain where I've been. It was clear from my last short return home that I'm sick and that I have had chemotherapy. There's a soft knit cap covering my bald head. I'm bones. But am I dying or healing? I don't know.

I am so happy to see our bedroom, the cheery minty-green walls, the framed tablecloth of embroidered birds (a trade I made with Nora for a hooked rug), Honey's lavender canvas doggy bed. I have to do something about that. Can't have Honey's empty doggy bed staring at me. But I like it. I like the idea that maybe she's around somewhere. Sunlight pours in. Peter and I are cozy together.

Graft-versus-host disease can come in horrible new forms. Because of the A-fib, I am also now more vulnerable to stroke— I have no idea how I acquired that information. Chemotherapy can cause my skin to produce melanomas. I can also, after all I've been through, get this killer AML all over again. A hornet's nest of possibilities. *Don't be scared of the treatment, be scared of leukemia.* The fear of all that battles an equally strong hope that the transplant worked. That I will survive.

My immune system is still severely compromised and will be for almost a year. I can't see babies or young children. Heather's little Rowan still can't visit. All eating restrictions are still in place. I can't go to the theater or a restaurant. No subways and so on and so forth.

I am living in a twilight world.

I am unable to walk without a rollator and even then not far. I don't have the strength or balance to stand alone. The hospital suggests that I spend five weeks in their rehab facility, but I can't bear to do that. We meet with two physical therapists who we can get through Medicare. I think I am allowed a few weeks' coverage. No one can come back from this enfeebled state in a few weeks. It's shocking how little government assistance helps.

We hire one of my physical therapists from the Weill Cornell rehab unit, Jessica Serpico, to come after work for an hour a day five days a week. No messing around. I'm in a hurry. I will bless her forever for not charging us, as the expression goes, an arm and a leg.

Jessica, twenty-six, is a wonder. Tall, confident, expert, fun, relaxed, and completely professional. A text arrives in the morning confirming our afternoon appointment. When she gets to the building, she texts, I'm here. She's always on time. No minute is wasted. She knows how to get every muscle in my seventy-three-year-old body back in shape.

She is right up there with Drs. Roboz and van Besien in helping me survive. Medicine has sent me home. She will put me back in the world.

My arms are still speckled red from a slightly low platelet count.

They start to clear, but then every so often, I sprout a few more spots. I check my arms daily, believing they are a warning sign of trouble. I show new ones to Peter, to Jessica. They assure me that this is normal.

Aside from the limitations of my body, I am not quite present mentally. I am anxious in company—which I don't want a lot of yet—uncertain. How much do I say about my illness? Do they want to hear it? Are they wondering what to ask? Feeling vulnerable and separate.

The anxiety of possibly getting deathly ill from any wandering germ makes me nervous too.

I have to relearn practically everything. I have no muscle tone. That's not an exaggeration. I build up my arms with five-pound weights that feel as if they weigh a ton.

I have to learn to stand up from a sitting position. First with the help of my hands, then without. More difficult, I have to get up from the floor. When I am on the floor trying to do this, I feel that I might just spend the rest of my life here. It's amazing to keep trying and trying and then suddenly be able to do it. Again and again and again.

I used to be able to walk over to the West Village in fifteen minutes. Now, with the help of a rollator and Jessica for safety, I manage to walk very slowly as far as the corner, where there is a beautiful flower shop. I have always loved its windows—explosions of color, of seasons, of holidays. I can't buy flowers. I'm still not allowed them, but they are all on display. Lilacs, anemones, ranunculi, tulips, daffodils, all miraculous not just because they are beautiful and delicate but because they are spring. They tell us we have survived another winter. I have survived a wicked winter.

Over the years I have seen many people on Tenth Street with

rollators and walkers. Old people. Sick people. I have felt sorry for them. I used to look away. I regret, am even appalled, by my previous lack of admiration and empathy. Now I am feeble and they are looking at me, or avoiding looking at me. I have to summon my nerve. I have to "own" it. *If you see my vulnerability,* I force myself to think, *well, I hope you respect my bravery.*

In a few weeks, I can make my way across the room holding on to walls, chairs, tables. "Furniture walking," Jessica calls it. There is a staircase in our duplex. It's not one of those spiral ones, but it does have a tricky turn in the middle. I can't imagine ever going up or down it. Fortunately, our apartment has a door out on both levels. To get from the bedroom to the kitchen, I exit the apartment, buzz for the elevator, and take it down a flight.

One day I suddenly start walking on my own.

Another day I look at the staircase and think, *I can go down that.* And I do. More amazingly, another day, I go up.

My body may be gaining strength, but I am not writing. Both my screenplay projects went south during my illness. I can't imagine sitting down in my office at my laptop and having any thoughts spill out. This is huge. I am a writer first. It's sanity and comfort. But it's gone. That big piece of me is in a boat caught in a current, drifting farther and farther away.

That I have Peter is a gigantic comfort. My brain may be a bit wonky, I may never write again, but how, at this moment in my life, did he and I find each other? I never lose the wonder of it.

Peter shrugs off the ordeal of the hospital, doesn't dwell on it, lets it go. I don't understand how he can, but he is sturdy emotionally. He says his resilience is from surviving the sudden death of his mother, from his medical training, and from having carried the weight for years of his patients' traumas. I need to talk about my trauma—melphalan still on my mind, my sense of awkwardness in the world, my fear of being outdoors alone—and he listens. But he notices and consistently reminds me of my progress. Every day I am eating more and getting physically stronger. Friends are coming to visit. I am enjoying them. Peter is loving it. He says that, during the weeks after I get out of the hospital, watching me heal, he is ecstatic.

I'm fortunate that Peter and my close friends took the trip with me, because they know where I've been. I am less alone because of that. There is a gulf between me and everyone else. Other friends and family and many business relationships that I really enjoy are on the other side of the moat. Trauma is isolating. I think about Nora. I can't understand how I am here and my sister is not. It's both guilt and confusion. It seems impossible that I survived and she didn't, but it appears to be happening, although I can't actually be sure of that.

I endlessly review the facts. A haplo-cord transplant didn't exist as an option when my sister was sick. Would she have undergone it if it had? And would she have survived? I'll never know. I wish she could have had the chance, the choice. She was determined not to suffer, had researched transplants then available and decided against them.

I am not my sister. My leukemia is not her leukemia. In addition to our illnesses being different under a microscope, our ways of being sick were different. I surrounded myself with friends. She preferred not to share. Sharing when you are famous is different and more overwhelming than sharing when you're not. She learned all the science and consulted many experts. She was a journalist; she began her career as a reporter. Journalists collect everything there is to know and make sense of it. I am not that. I write mainly from inside. I learned as little as possible. Sisterhood can be muddy— where she ended and I began was not always clear. Nora always said that we "shared half a brain"—but when we were sick, we were most clearly not alike.

I know that trying to get well from leukemia ate up every ounce of me, mentally and physically. I needed every morsel of friendship for sustenance. Even though Nora was gone, she was with me on this journey through the friends who sustained me. Linda—with me almost every day—worked for Nora first, then for both of us. Jessie and Jon were Nora's friends. They became mine soon after Nora died. Meredith and I met thirty-five years ago because of Nora. "You have to meet my sister," Nora told her when Jerry and I moved to LA.

And Peter. My sister set me up with him when I was eighteen years old.

Slowly healing now, I begin to miss life. There are small pleasures I am craving. Soon, if I stay well, I can hang out with a girlfriend at Buvette, have tarte tatin and a cappuccino. Peter and I can have dinner with friends in a restaurant. I can go to my beloved neighborhood Il Cantinori. We can take long walks in the Village. I cannot wait to go back to the theater. I want to take a subway. In the meantime, I am happy simply to watch Wimbledon this year, to cheer for Nadal, to sit with Peter on our couch and eat dinner on our piano bench. Maybe Jessie and Bryan will watch with us.

I show up at Dr. van Besien's clinic twice a week, then once a week, then every two weeks. When I first arrive with the rollator, managing it like a pro, his staff praise me wildly. I am so proud of myself. VB reassures me about the red speckles too. My hearing has been hit badly from the treatment. "What?" is now my favorite word. I mention this, and VB says, "On your last visit, you asked me 'What?' twice." *Good grief,* I think, *he notices everything.* He is such a careful doctor. I decide to wait a bit before dealing with my hearing loss. Less medicine right now is better.

In several months, he tells me, I will have to be vaccinated for everything again. Baby shots—measles, polio, the works. All my childhood immunities are gone.

"Are you writing?" he asks.

"No," I say.

I don't add *Never again,* but it's what I think.

VB has been reducing my pill intake. Even mentioning this now makes me teary with joy. I don't know how he even tracks so many, many pills, what they can do and not do, and their interactions. These pills have been my torturers. And he is cutting them back.

The few remaining are all tolerable, mainly because there are just a few. Peter puts them on a little saucer for me every morning. I take them easily now with yogurt.

I begin to find out more about Dr. van Besien. I google him for the first time and then ask him lots of questions. He is the youngest of ten children. He became a doctor, he explains in the modest way that is his style, because everyone in his family was either an architect or a doctor and "I didn't have the talent to be an architect." He speaks five languages: English, French, Dutch, German, Spanish. He went to medical school in Belgium, received an advanced degree in the Netherlands, then did fellowships in hematology/oncology in Bruges and at Indiana University. He has worked in various U.S. hospitals: he was on the faculty of the transplant program at MD Anderson in Houston and directed the transplant and lymphoma program at the University of Chicago before running the stem cell/bone marrow transplant program at Weill Cornell. The language of transplants...I don't know what half the words mean. It's not just that he can order coffee in different languages—he can practice medicine in foreign languages. To me—I studied French for several years and my accent is still so bad it's practically a comedy routine—this is mind-blowing. He has researched and experimented with lifesaving cures for blood cancers, including the haplo-cord transplant that saved my life. He enjoys his patients and speaks of them with such respect. "Emergency medicine could never be for me," he says. With transplants, he can follow his patients for years. He is very busy researching cures and saving lives, yet he finds time to read my novel *Siracusa*. He knows who I am. Not simply because he reengineered my bone marrow. He takes the trouble to know my brain and heart.

Text, me to Dr. Roboz, June 5, 2018:

Just to let you know I'm feeling stronger and happier every day.

E-mail, me to Dr. Roboz (who is at a conference in Stockholm) after another bone marrow biopsy, June 16, 2018:

VB said my morphology was great on my bone marrow and there was nothing to worry about. This was on Thursday. I asked him twice, was he absolutely sure, and he said yes. There were a few genetics that weren't in yet but there was absolutely nothing to worry about. I have never been so relieved. I sure hope you agree.

In spite of googling it, I have no idea what *morphology* means or why I used it so confidently in an e-mail.

From Dr. Roboz to me:

> Yes! I hope you are wearing your "Don't Worry, Be Happy" T shirt! See you soon and congrats. Am flying home tomorrow.

Me to Dr. Roboz, June 28:

> Just to say my blood counts are fantastic. I can climb the stairs in my apartment and walk remarkable distances.

After an appointment with VB, Peter and I stop in at the other end of the third floor at Dr. Roboz's clinic, just to say hi. I mention to her, with some joy, that I'm not getting horrible rashes. Horrible rashes are a major symptom of graft-versus-host disease.

"Shush," says Dr. Roboz, as if the witches will hear.

Gail M. is moving out of our building. She, Marti, and Moki are relocating to Nyack. How is this possible? Who would leave Tenth Street? I am so sad about it. A year or so before my transplant, Marti, a social worker and professor in the NYU School of Social Work, retired, and recently Gail M. cut back on her patients. Gail M. knows everyone in our building. I corralled her when I was sick, but I think I'm only one of many who depend on her wisdom and spirit. Still finding it hard to rejoice in my new health, I have continued to bring my dark worries to her.

"It could still all go up in smoke," I tell her. Then, despairing at my inability to be more positive, I say, "I can't be in the moment."

Gail tells me she doesn't know what that means. "Terror is the background of noise one lives with while being in life," she says.

In other words, it's just there. It's inescapable.

I learned that lesson early. I learned it by living with my mother, who terrorized me. From eleven on I was frightened every night, by my parents screaming and fighting, by my alcoholic mother beset with demons and spreading them around, mad rants, doors slammed. I put my fingers in my ears, diluted liquor bottles, pulled pillows over my head, hid under blankets, under beds. Every day I worried about what might occur that night, and something always did. The anatomy of what happens to each of us is shadowed and affected by what came before, and I was conditioned as a child to live with fear and worry. My brain knows that place. It gravitates toward it no matter how bright the lights or the love and health.

One of the special things about my friendship with Julia is that it has taught me that not everyone worries all the time. She doesn't. Julia is sunny. She is untraumatized. Richard has been slowly diminishing, the evils of Parkinson's—he falls again and again. Lately he breaks one limb and then another. It's been brutal, and she suffers too, but anxiety is not home for her. Terror isn't a childhood friend. She can experience terror and let it go. But I am conditioned. My brain gives terror a home.

By July I am seeing VB only every three weeks. Every three weeks! I walk confidently into the hospital. I suppose I could even run if I had to. My hair is starting to exist. Short and cool. Eugene does something with it. Lisa and Marie tell me I look like Jean Seberg, the actress in French movies. Got to love my friends who tell me that. At seventy-four now (a birthday I never expected to see), I look like Jean Seberg.

Since my diagnosis in March 2017, a year and four months ago, I have been hospitalized or at the hospital a minimum of once a week, often getting transfused. No transfusions now. I am producing my own healthy blood. I am over the moon with my normalcy.

After my appointment with VB on July 26, Peter and I walk to the other end of the hall to say hi to Dr. Roboz and her team: Natalie, Evgeny, and Marie. Whoa, wow, huge smiles, hugs. They are happy to see me. Proud of my health.

Text, me to Dr. Roboz, night of July 26, 2018:

I am looking at all my texts to you during the transplant. It's overwhelming to me that you pulled me through, and through the darkest. "Give me 48 hours," you said, "and if it's working, give me another 48." And here I am climbing stairs, my taste buds are back, my counts rising, and everything coming back. It was wonderful to see you today (and all the divine people who work with you). VB has been fantastic— he is spectacular, you both have this amazing intuitive thing— I felt so cared for. Thank you is inadequate, but I'll say it anyway. Thank you. Delia

E-mail from Elyse Martin, August 20, 2018:

Hi there,

Hope all is well with you. Good thing you never pursued me as a stem cell donor. I went to the hematologist today with a slightly elevated white and leukocyte count. She's pretty sure I have CLL. I guess our connection keeps getting more interesting.

XO,

Elyse

Receiving this e-mail stunned me.

CLL is a mild form of leukemia. People who have it can live for years and years without even getting treatment for it, but it is leukemia. I remember Elyse's generosity in offering to be my donor. Dr. Roboz and Meredith counseled against testing her, and what a relief they did. Suppose Elyse and I had matched and she had been my donor?

Elyse and I continue to check in with each other. Her illness remains under control, I'm thrilled to say, and not only that, she falls madly in love.

*I*n September I am cleared to fly. After a transplant, restrictions are in place for at least a year. VB does not think flying is as dangerous as going to movies or theaters or sitting in a restaurant or, especially, being around children. The air in the plane, he tells me, is circulated. We take disinfectants to wipe down the trays. Many instructions are given to Peter's kids about how I can't be around anyone with a sniffle. It's no way to get to know a grand-child, worrying any minute she might get too close. No way either to make friends with Peter's grown kids. We have a wonderful dinner with Meredith and her partner, Steve. I'm growing attached to San Rafael. The takeout Chinese chicken salad at Magnolia Park Kitchen right near our apartment is scrumptious. The cappuccino at Aroma is made with Graffeo coffee beans, which are excellent. There is an extraordinary farmers' market on Sunday on a huge field near the Marin County Civic Center—more varieties of peaches and plums than I have ever seen, all available to sample, plus my beloved petite Sun Gold tomatoes, varieties of exotic vegetables and lettuces, baked goods, local butter. The civic center itself is a remarkable structure designed by Frank Lloyd Wright.

Peter buys me a baseball glove and we start playing catch in the park.

We have been having a nice time when, after improving steadily since May, I wake up one morning with a migraine.

I've never had a migraine but I know instantly from the drilling pain piercing my eye that a migraine is what it is. A migraine is viciously unmistakable. Mine doesn't go away at night. It lasts days. I throw up in the car. My illness up to now, debilitating and terrorizing as it is, has never been painful. Migraines, as anyone who has had one can tell you, are brutal.

I call Dr. Kurth, my internist, and she prescribes a heavy-duty drug. When I lie down on the bed after taking it, the ceiling spins. The experience is almost as scary as the migraine.

The migraines come and go during our trip west. I think it's graft-versus-host disease. Peter disagrees. He says it's simply my body responding to its "new self." This right here is a big difference between us. He is positive, and I am not. I'm suspicious, he's trusting. I'm scared, he's confident. My body is not rejecting anything, he says, it's adjusting.

Peter won't ever go negative with me. He simply refuses. And he's calm about all my anxieties. He won't go into that rattling place and he tries not to let me go. He always pulls me back. I don't know how he can be like that—I get anxious so quickly.

When I get back to New York, Dr. Kurth ups my Zoloft, which I have been on ever since this transplant began. And by the end of September, the migraines have stopped paying visits.

I am missing Wales, pining to see Julia and Richard. Richard is eighty-eight now and his Parkinson's is accelerating. He broke a femur last year. Julia has gotten out of bed in the middle of the night and found him sprawled on the stairs. I don't know how many more visits we will have. We decide to go.

The flight, overnight from JFK, is on time, but it is raining in Dublin where we change planes, and the long walk in the cold under an awning to wherever the hell we are going—another terminal, the connecting flight to Bristol—is daunting. I suppose I should have ordered a wheelchair, but I preferred to worry myself into a state and then be proud I could do the trek.

Julia and Richard's farmhouse, called Whitebrook, feels like Brigadoon, a mythical town that appears only one day every one hundred years. It's ancient, unchanging, not visible as we drive the curvy road and then suddenly, as if out of a mist, there it is, set back, a simple white box of a house bordered by low ancient stone walls. Their dog Jelly Bean waits in the driveway. A few chickens are on the loose. Richard is not well enough to come down the walk to greet us.

Awful illnesses shred our modesty, our poise, our ability to present ourselves. Yet we are, not always but often, still who we are inside, and Richard, crumpled in a chair, his voice faint, remains wise, comforting, honest, and a force. He's not frightened about death, he confides one afternoon when it's just the two of us. Jerry said the same. I don't understand that. Richard is at peace, which is different from what I felt. My wanting to die was desperate.

In spite of his illness—the jangle of the alarm alerting us that it's time for his pills, and the sadness and worry of watching how difficult it is for him to stand, to move even the shortest distances— in spite of that, our all being together is still soothing, even joyful. Richard shares his sadness that their daughter, Poppy, is moving with her husband, Sam, and their two toddlers to Sydney. They completely understand her need to travel, even relocate. We commiserate. Poppy and Sam are young, they're figuring it out; their need for discovery has urgency. We want comfort. We want simply to reexperience the happiness we've found for as long as we can.

This visit is a bit of the same, and the same feels precious and fleeting.

We stay in their barn, which is cozy and in shouting distance of the house. Julia arranges two massages for me that, she says, when she had one, made her feel like a "box of birds." No one talks like Julia, no one advises like Richard. My energy is low, and the five-hour time adjustment is difficult. We all play bridge. Julia and Peter take long walks with Jelly. Peter loves the beauty of Wales as much as I do. Julia and I hang out in the kitchen. I eat chocolate-covered ginger biscuits and crumpets soaked in butter. We talk about Richard falling, the stress and terror of living with that, Julia's novel, friends of mine she has met, friends of hers I have met. Whether I'll ever write again. No, I say, that part of my life is over.

"It can't be," says Julia.

"It is," I insist.

I don't ask the one thing that worries me. This place is home to me almost as much as Tenth Street. Conversation, friendship, laughter, and understanding are my favorite sports, and, for me, the game is played better here than it is anywhere else. I can't drive on the roads; I can't figure out how to get an egg out of a chicken coop, although I can manage the Aga. But Jerry's ashes are here. Why are a Bronx-bred Jewish man's ashes scattered in the green fields of Wales? They are here because this is where we were our happiest and best selves. So I don't ask: *Will you move from Whitebrook when you lose Richard?* It is clear, tragically, that this loss will happen one day soon.

No one can truly know the answer to the question, What will you do when you lose the person you love?

But will Julia not only sell Whitebrook but also, to be near Poppy, move to Australia? Australia. That's the other side of the moon. I can't bear to think ahead, but I must be feeling stronger, because I am thinking ahead.

February 2019. One year since my stem cell transplant.

Jessie has directed and cowritten a musical, *Alice by Heart*, that is opening at a lovely off-Broadway theater uptown near Fifty-Seventh Street. It's about a young girl named Alice who has to take shelter in a London tube station during the bombing in World War II. She finds her spirit, bravery, and a way back to life through the storybook she knows by heart, *Alice in Wonderland*. In its own way, the musical is a trip through a tunnel of love.

Peter and I bump into VB just outside the elevator when we're on our way to his clinic. May I go to the theater? I ask him. It's a small shiny newish theater and very clean (is there such a thing?), I believe I tell him. Yes, he says.

God. How amazing. I am going out. I am going to sit with a large group of people and share an experience. We will watch a show. Jessie's opening night. Or is it my opening night? It's her show, but it is my coming-out party. When Peter and I walk through the crowd—a crowd!—and into the theater and see her standing across the aisle, it's hard to know who is happier, although she is more nervous. And she looks beautiful, absolutely glowing.

We both tear up. She starts to explain to people she's with why we are so emotional, but it's too complicated, too personal. So she just keeps saying, "I can't believe you're here."

Heather and I resume coffee dates that go on forever. And shortly after that, she brings Rowan, her adorable two-year-old, over for Sunday breakfast. Last viewing—he was at Peter and my party to celebrate our marriage. I can't hug him—I might catch something—but I make him pancakes, which he loves. He plays hide-and-seek with Peter, and every time he hides, he shouts, "Here I am!"

My appointments with Dr. van Besien are now every three months, and I need to work out with Jessica only two days a week. My hair is bizarre. It grows in thick, that's the good part, but wild with rippling curls and sort of a wiry texture but soft. It's strange and uncontrollable. Meredith calls it "happy hair." Before I was sick, I wrote a recurring hashtag on Twitter called #TheHairReport based on the idea that women don't care about the weather, they only care what the weather will do to their hair. My hair right now has a mind of its own, regardless of weather. I'm trying to adjust. *Okay,* I think, *weird, wild hair forever. That's what it will be.* Eugene still bosses it around, but I think it's a bigger challenge.

*A*t an appointment with Dr. van Besien sometime in the spring, he says this: "Two years from your transplant is when the AML is likely to come back."

Two years. That's February 2020. I didn't realize that. I thought the transplant was a cure. My heart flips. I go silent. I have only nine months. I don't say anything else at the appointment and I don't mention how much it upsets me to Peter, who is there with me. I don't know why I don't, but I don't. I begin to count the days, every day in 2019 brings me closer to February 2020 when I'm at risk again. I am so happy now, I can't bear to think it will come back. We fly to California to visit Peter's kids and grandkids and then drive down to LA, where I see everyone I love. Peter and I go with Deena and her husband, Marty, to a Dodger game. We are in the sun, and since I have had chemotherapy, the sun feels brutal—there is some scientific reason for this—so I last only five innings but eat a delicious frank. Hot dogs and ball games, there's nothing better. We hang out with Phil, Jill, and their kids, Fia and Emmett. I decide to send Honey's dog bed to Fia for her cat, Wayne Sanchez.

There is a shadow over all this because next year is coming, and perhaps my illness will be back. One day, lounging in Peter's office, I tell him how much what VB said haunts me. Peter swivels in his chair to face me. "VB didn't say that. VB said, 'After two years it's unlikely your leukemia will ever come back.'"

"You are completely wrong," I say.

We have an argument about it. "I heard it," I tell him again and again.

"That's not what he said," says Peter. "He said that after two years, your disease is unlikely to ever come back."

To prove Peter wrong, I check with VB.

Peter is right. I took VB's words and flipped them. Positive to negative. I carried the information around like a precious fear, letting it haunt and taint every renewal. My hearing. Of course, my awful hearing. I should have said to VB, "What?" I should have said, *"What?"* Instead, I took doom and ran with it.

One morning shortly after straightening this out, I sit down at the computer and type into the search bar *Petfinder.com.*

I miss Honey terribly. Miss the sound of her clambering up the stairs, miss her cuddling her squeaky toy gorillas, which now occupy a shelf in my office, miss her fixations on me when she wanted a treat, miss all the love, action, and conversation she brought to my life. Peter has never had a dog. Peter would love a dog.

Combing rescue sites for dogs is addictive. It begins to eat my life. In fact, the second I go to Petfinder.com, I know normal life is over until this problem gets solved. Of course, I haven't had much of a normal life lately, so this is a welcome diversion. That I am doing this also tells me I believe I will live.

I want a female (I think they are easier than males) that Peter and I can take on a plane when we go to California, so she has to be under fifteen pounds, and I am not wild for Pekingese or Chihuahuas, of which many are available. Also, I want an older dog. I am older, my dog should be too.

A friend of mine puts me in touch with Tiffany Lacey at Animal Haven in New York City, and she is great. She will end up getting two of my friends fantastic dogs when I pass her name on. But she has nothing now that meets my requirements.

One day, in the lobby of my building, I bump into Lucy.

Lucy is a small white Havanese, as was Honey. I am crazy for Havanese, because they are funny. I can't actually explain how, but it's true, and I am sure everyone who has a Havanese knows that. I ask Lucy's owner, Ann, where she got Lucy. "Peace Love Havanese," she says. "Near Woodstock, New York."

Peace Love Havanese. Could there be a more perfect name?

Of course I would find the solution to this problem right in my own lobby.

Daisy, my first pup, was a rescue. Honey was not. There is no guilt like the guilt of explaining that you actually paid money for a dog, with all the dogs needing rescue, but I have, and at that moment I suspect I will again.

I look at the website. Clear, smart, friendly, with excellent information about the breed and full of pictures of happy owners cuddling their pets. We call Diane Moshe, the breeder, and have a lovely chat. She used to, in an earlier life, live in Brooklyn, then Greenwich Village, which I take as a very good sign. I ask her if she by any chance has an older female who is done having her pups and can be adopted. "Heidi," she says. But, she explains, Heidi is a difficult dog. Diane isn't sure Heidi could adjust to city life. We can come and meet her if we want.

I hang up and Peter and I discuss whether we should rent a car, drive up, and meet Heidi. We have friends who live nearby, in Kingston. We could stop there and make it a day. *Why not?* we're thinking when the phone rings. It's Diane. She also has another dog, Charlotte. Charlotte is six months old. Diane had been planning to keep Charlotte to breed her but she's too small. Charlotte, she says, is perfect for us. Why don't we meet Charlotte too?

She sends a picture. Charlotte is black with white paws, a white belly, and a little white beard. Her fur falls like a curtain to the floor, and with her mouth open and tongue peeking out, she looks suitably goofy. Already I'm thinking, *Okay, if we die, whom will we leave her to?* I obviously have to plan for this. Charlotte will outlive me and probably Peter. Death is the shadow, even with something joyful. But that is normal now. That is old-age normal. Within a minute I come up with at least four friends who might take her.

We're on our way to Woodstock to meet Heidi and Charlotte that Sunday.

We pull into the driveway of Diane's homey wood-framed house with a peaked roof, and the second we do, we are greeted with the joyful racket of barking Havanese. We are obviously in the right place.

Diane's living room is cozy with a lovely fire burning in the fireplace. There are three litters nursing in the next room. The puppies are tiny, each a little smaller than my hand. A couple of older dogs race around us. Outside, against a sliding glass door to a deck, several pups jump, aching to get in.

It's an easy choice. Diane puts Heidi in my lap. Heidi jumps off and tears away. Diane puts Charlotte in my lap. Charlotte snuggles while she licks Peter's hand. She's instantly ours.

Diane will have her spayed, and we will pick her up next Sunday.

Diane suggests we change her name if we want. But Charlotte the spider in *Charlotte's Web* is one of my favorite characters in all fiction. She saves Wilbur the pig's life, and at the end of the book, after she dies, author E. B. White declares, "It is not often that someone comes along who is a true friend and a good writer. Charlotte was both."

That is all I've aspired to. True friend and good writer. It seems only right that Charlotte should be our dog's name.

Charlotte turns out to be a super-snuggly pup, although on walks she moves very quickly. If you see a handsome seventy-plus man sprinting down Tenth Street with a nine-pound black-and-white ball of fur, that's Peter and Charlotte.

I would like to meet my donor. After a year, it's permitted, if both people want to. I am allowed to meet the adult donor but not the baby (or the mother of the baby) whose cord blood is now my blood. I know only that the baby was a boy.

Who is this person who saved my life? Where does she or he live, what nationality, what language? How does she or he spend her or his days? Why did the donor do it? It never crossed my mind to give my stem cells to save a random person whose name, age, religion, and politics are irrelevant to me. I had never heard of a bone marrow bank until it came up with my sister's illness.

I tell Dr. van Besien I would like to meet the donor, and within a few weeks I get an e-mail along with her release from Be the Match: "Sign your name below to show that you have read this form and want to share your personal information with your donor or recipient."

In clear, legible handwriting, she has signed *Casey McClaine*. She has filled in her phone number, e-mail, and location: Niceville, Florida.

Niceville? My donor lives in a town called Niceville? I simply can't believe it. How magical. How perfect.

Where exactly is Niceville? Here's what it says in Google.

Niceville is a town in Okaloosa County, Florida, United States, located near Eglin Air Force Base on Boggy Bayou that opens into Choctawhatchee Bay. The population was 11,684 at the 2000 census. The 2010 census population for Niceville was 12,749.

Okaloosa, Boggy Bayou, Choctawhatchee—beautiful words conjuring up misty magical landscapes, exotic blooms, large feathered birds. I would move there just for the words. Simply, it's the Florida Gulf Coast.

E-mail from me to Casey McClaine, September 17, 2019:

Dear Casey,

I wanted to thank you for being my match for a bone marrow transplant.

Because of you I am alive …

Really, I can barely think how to begin to thank you for this gift. But I would at least like to do it by phone if that's okay with you.

I live in New York City.

I have your phone number but didn't want to surprise you by calling cold.

Please let me know if phoning is okay, and when might be a good time.

With all my gratitude,

Delia Ephron

I don't hear back for five days. Which is odd, I think. I discuss it with forty-five or so people. I text her. Maybe she's more into texting. Most of the world is now.

Text from me to Casey, September 23, 2019:

> Hi Casey,
>
> I'm your bone marrow transplant recipient. I emailed you a week ago, didn't hear back. Want to call and thank you. You are the reason I'm alive. If it's okay to phone, let me know. And when might be a good time. If you'd rather I didn't phone, please know how grateful I am.
>
> Delia Ephron

Text from Casey to me, September 26, 2019:

> Delia, thank you for contacting me. I apologize for the late response. I've been on vacation. I'd love to hear from you. I am available at any point tomorrow and during the day on Saturday, Sunday, and Monday. If any one of these works for you then I'll be hearing from you soon! I appreciate your gratitude and willingness to reach out to me!
>
> Casey

She is obviously both gracious and literate. Although, after I hear how complicated, even daunting, it is to be a transplant donor, I suspect donating stem cells attracts a bright, sensitive, and intelligent group.

I'm trying to think if I've ever made a call as momentous as this. My first conversation with Peter was weighted with possibility. But this call to Casey has no bearing on my future. It's a thank-you to her for giving me a future.

I call and she doesn't answer, and then I get a text that she is held up at the grocery store. And then she calls. She couldn't be nicer.

I flood her with gratitude and then ask her how this all came about.

She was twenty-five when she registered with DKMS: We Delete Blood Cancer, an international bone marrow donor center originating in Germany. As I mentioned before, all these bone marrow registries around the world cooperate. Twenty-five years old. To me, that's young to realize you can play a part in saving lives. She was twenty-seven when she donated her stem cells to me. She grew up in St. Louis. Her mother, who is a nurse, told Casey about it. "I registered because I thought everyone should. If someone else has the opportunity, they should do it too."

She sent her application and half a cup of her saliva to DKMS. "I never got anything back. A year and a half went by. I was actually wondering about it and tried looking into it to see if I was in the registry, to no avail, a few weeks to a month before I learned that I had matched with you."

E-mail to Casey from DKMS:

> Hi Casey,
> Hope all is well. Thank you so much for registering as a bone marrow donor. I called earlier and left you a voice mail with some good news—the patient's doctors have selected you as a patient's matching donor and that patient is ready to receive a transplant. At this time, they are asking if you would be willing to donate to the patient.

"Yes," she answered.

She was told that the procedure was "innovative."

"You are invited to participate in an innovative therapy plan for a recipient with acute myelogenous leukemia. The recipient will receive a haploidentical unrelated bone marrow or peripheral blood stem cell (PBSC) transplant followed by a cord blood transplant."

Could she have possibly understood what this meant? I've been through it and I barely do. But she did, actually, and added, "The implication of 'innovative' was fascinating to me, as the research surrounding the success of the transplant could potentially be beneficial to others in the future." The last line of the e-mail: "You will not benefit from participating in this innovative therapy."

That's a literal interpretation: "You will not benefit." I assume it means monetarily? Maybe physically? What about the more spiritual reward of being emotionally generous? Or saving a life?

There was a clock ticking on her donation. It was December, and my transplant was scheduled for February. Casey said, "I was sent a lot of paperwork to fill out, print, scan and return. All sorts of personal information about my health." Then her blood was drawn at a local clinic. "It was analyzed to be sure I was healthy," she said. During this time she was, she said, "excited."

After she passed that hurdle, they sent her a plane ticket. She flew from Destin–Fort Walton Beach Airport to Atlanta, changed planes, and flew to Washington, DC.

In DC she went to Georgetown University Hospital and had a physical. They put her up in the hotel next to the hospital. She took Ubers and Lyfts and sent the receipts for reimbursement. A day later they flew her back to Florida.

Then she received final approval.

Many donors, I am told, crash out during this time, either

because they don't pass the physical requirements or because they change their minds.

The preparation for the actual extraction of her stem cells was rigorous. She was FedExed Neupogen, packed in ice, with the instruction "Transfer to the refrigerator as soon as possible (a vegetable drawer is ideal)." Neupogen is a drug that stimulates the growth of white blood cells. A nurse showed up at her house every day for four days to give her a shot of it. There were cautions. Avoid certain drugs for two weeks before the donation: aspirin, Motrin, Advil. Two days before, take over-the-counter calcium; four days before, avoid alcohol. The day before, drink plenty of fluids and avoid caffeine. The morning of, drink fluids, avoid caffeine, eat a healthy protein-rich breakfast, and wear loose-fitting clothes.

Donating stem cells appears to be quite an undertaking. Flying back and forth, getting medical exams, spending your own cash and filing later for reimbursement, filling out paperwork, avoiding this, consuming that. Getting shots. This is bravery. This is inconvenience. This is serious good works. This is kindness.

In the middle of February, she was flown back to Washington, this time with her boyfriend, and put up for two nights at the hotel connected to Georgetown University Hospital.

She sent me a photo of herself having her stem cells harvested. She's in a blue T-shirt, lying under the covers in a hospital bed. Her long black hair is pulled back from her young and innocent face. There are two IVs hooked up to her and to a large, complicated-looking machine with all sorts of knobs and dials. One IV takes her blood and sends it to the machine that harvests her stem cells; the other IV gives her back what's left. Casey looks a tiny bit dazed. She's smiling, yes, she's definitely happy, but also vulnerable. I can see as well as tell from talking to her that she is a spirited young woman. I hope she gave me some of that energy. She lay there for five and a half hours while they harvested her stem cells to give me life.

Casey and I have stayed in touch. "It's taken me pretty long to decide what I've wanted to do," she said. In 2019 she enrolled at the University of Florida and will graduate with a degree in Health Education and Behavior and become a CHES (certified health education specialist).

"When I got your e-mail," said Casey, "I was incredibly happy. I was floored that I had the chance to help somebody. I was curious as to whether you would want to reach out to me. I would jump at the chance. To know this life that I helped save."

*L*ife slowly becomes more normal. I feel secure on my own. Peter flies to Denver to visit friends and drives to Moab to take a river-rafting trip. He misses his red-rock canyons. My sister Hallie comes to stay with me. To get one of our favorite childhood things, onion patty melts, we walk ten blocks to the restaurant and ten blocks back. A triumph.

While Peter is away I also have dinner with Eric, a composer of musical theater who lives in our building. At dinner I tell him a couple of stories of the strange events in North Carolina, of discovering things that I had already written. After dinner I give him my novel *The Lion Is In* and suggest that it might make a good musical. I say this without thinking.

He reads it and agrees, and soon we are meeting weekly at my dining-room table to find the story, the structure, and the songs. Eric and I eat a lot of popcorn while he schools me in how to write the book of a musical. Something challenging to try to master. Something new. Eric is easygoing and so smart. And he lives four flights down. It could not be better. How perfect that I am adapting this novel whose premise I dreamed when Jerry and Nora first got sick. It calmed me then. It's back now to coax me into the happy world of my imagination.

Like that, I'm writing again.

*I*n February 2020, I have my two-year appointment with Dr. van Besien. Two years since the transplant. We sit in clinic room 26. "This is a social visit," says Dr. van Besien. "Now your chances of getting leukemia again are the same as mine and I've never had it."

I almost dance out of his clinic. Peter and I make a stop at the other end of the third floor. We catch Dr. Roboz and her gang in the hall-way. Dr. Roboz is rushing off to do a European radio show. I burst out with my happy news. Dr. Roboz beams. She gives me a hug. Evgeny calls me a rock star. For sure I am that. They fuss over me.

I can take the subway. We ride the Q train home.

My neighborhood is mine again. I visit Ron at the antiques store; we chat about this and that, our usual, what theater he's recently seen. I eat grilled calamari at a normal crowded hour at my beloved Il Cantinori. Frank, who owns it, is delighted to see me. Every-where I go, I get greeted with happiness and cheers for my bravery. It's lovely but I don't think I was brave. I was a captive on a no-exit journey. One way only. And, simply, I was fortunate that I didn't die. I got my disease at a time of scientific discovery. I had great medicine and great love.

And luck. That was a big part of my story. Is *luck* another word for *miracle?* I don't know, but the amount of luck I had almost tips it into that zone. Luck that my internet broke, that I wrote about it, that Peter read about it and wrote to me. Luck that I found Dr. Roboz, that she was already in my medical life when I got sick, that my six-month regular appointment with her was randomly scheduled within a week or so of my getting AML. In my treatment I benefited from a confluence of events. Confluence—a miraculous coming together. It's a word Peter and I used repeatedly in our first e-mails to each other. When I got sick, there were ten new drugs for AML (including CPX-351) after, as Dr. Roboz puts it, "years of nothing." This coincided with the development of the haplo-cord transplant (the idea of combining adult donor blood with umbilical cord blood), a procedure specially for people who don't have perfect matches, which I didn't. And for the first time, there was the notion that transplants could be done on people like me, over seventy, old people.

My friends were part of this journey. They were, one and all, extraordinary.

And Peter was there, most especially, steadfast through it all.

A lot of good fortune wrapped around very bad fortune.

Having come back from the brink, I don't lose a sense of wonder both that I've been there and that now I am miraculously not.

Most happily, I am writing again. Every day I go into my office and sit down at my laptop and write.

Soon I am writing this.

Acknowledgments

In April 2020, just after New York City began its COVID lockdown, I asked Julia Baylis to go through e-mails, texts, and drafts in my computer and phone and find everything related to my life between October 2015 and February 2018. Julia pulled together everything and organized it by date into five gigantic loose-leaf binders, which became the basis for this book. Without her help, I could never have written it.

Everything in this book is accurate to the best of my memory and research. I have done my best to get the medical facts correct. Very occasionally, some details are scrambled to protect the privacy of the person I am writing about. Jerry did not have a relative named Lulu. I made up that name because I did not remember the woman's name, but the story is true.

All the e-mails and texts reprinted are as originally written, although occasionally cut down. I thank everyone for permitting me to run them and for allowing me to use their names. The *New York Times* op-ed about Verizon was longer when it was originally published, and it is slightly altered/improved, I hope, as I never stop fussing with things I write.

Thank you to all my dearest friends who took this life journey with me and then read my drafts and gave me notes and discussed my manuscript with me endlessly: Sarah Dunn, Deena

Goldstone, Julia Gregson, Jessie Nelson, Natasha Gregson Wagner, and Meredith White. Also mountainous thanks to Jon LaPook, whose kindness, wisdom, and friendship helped me find my way through the fray. To Teodolinda Diaz—more familiarly known as Linda Diaz—I would not be here without you. To Eric Schorr for his careful read and for getting me back into writing. To my building for being a Village paradise. To all my friends, and some relatives, who also got me through the tunnel: Alice Abarbanel, Rachel Bernstein, Heather Chaplin, Jill Cordes, Stephen Earle, Mitchell Gross, Anna Harari, Lauren Hobbs, Rebecca Kurth, Kate Lear, Joel Mason, Gail Monaco, Helen Shim, Eugene Smith, Sue Territo, and Luc Verschueren. To Elena Seibert for her beautiful photos. To my wonderful sisters Hallie Ephron and Amy Ephron.

To Nora, who brought so much joy and adventure into my life and who also brought me Peter, Meredith, Linda, Jessie, and Jon.

To my brilliant and caring doctors Dr. Gail Roboz and Dr. Koen van Besien, my deepest gratitude. I don't understand how you do what you do, but thank goodness you are so mind-bendingly remarkable at it.

To Jessica Serpico, PT DTP, my physical therapist, who finished the work of bringing me back into the world.

To everyone at New York Presbyterian / Weill Cornell Medical Center who took such good care of me. To the amazing nurses on Ten West. To Mia Glassberg, who got me my six-thousand-plus pages of inpatient hospital records so quickly and always looked after me—thank you.

To Casey McClaine for her generous heart.

To my brother-in-law Nick Pileggi, for his generosity in providing a peaceful place to spend the winter to write.

For the friendship, wisdom, and joy of Richard Gregson, my dear friend, who died on August 21, 2019.

To Lynn Nesbit, the most gifted agent. Years now we have been together. Always compassionate, supportive, smart, clear, utterly trustworthy. A guiding force. To Claire Conrad at Janklow & Nesbit UK for her care in finding homes for my story in the larger world.

To my editor Judy Clain at Little, Brown. A more gifted guide/improver/champion of this book could not be imagined. And to everyone at Little, Brown who worked with me on this book: Sabrina Callahan, Anna de la Rosa, Elece Green, Michelle Figueroa, Jayne Yaffe Kemp, Miya Kumangai, Tracy Roe, Craig Young. And for my beautiful cover, thank you, Lauren Harms.

To Jerry, my compass, for our love and our memories.

To Peter, who was with me every single minute. Every day is magical because you are in it. All my love.

About the Author

Delia Ephron is a best-selling author, screenwriter, essayist, and playwright. Her novels include the *New York Times* best seller *Siracusa* and *The Lion Is In*. She has written books of essays—most recently *Sister Mother Husband Dog (Etc.)*—as well as books of humor, including *How to Eat Like a Child*, and books for children and young adults. Her movie credits include *You've Got Mail*, *The Sisterhood of the Traveling Pants*, *This Is My Life*, *Michael*, and *Hanging Up* (based on her novel). Her play, *Love, Loss, and What I Wore*, written with her sister Nora Ephron (based on the book by Ilene Beckerman), ran for two years off Broadway and has been performed all over the world.